Guide to Physical Security Planning & Response

For Hospitals, Medical, & Long Term Care Facilities

Includes Comprehensive Section on Evacuation Best Practices

All-Hazards Planning & Response - Templates - Best Practices

Mary Russell, Jim Kendig, & Don Philpott

Published by

Government Training Inc.™

ISBN: 978-1-937246-68-6

About the Publisher – Government Training Inc.™

Government Training Inc. provides worldwide training, publishing and consulting to government agencies and contractors that support government in areas of business and financial management, acquisition and contracting, physical and cyber security and intelligence operations. Our management team and instructors are seasoned executives with demonstrated experience in areas of Federal, State, Local and DoD needs and mandates.

For more information on the company, its publications and professional training, go to www.GovernmentTrainingInc.com.

For information regarding permissions, write to:
Government Training Inc.
Rights and Contracts Department
5372 Sandhamn Place
Longboat Key, Florida 34228
don.dickson@GovernmentTrainingInc.com

ISBN: 978-1-937246-68-6

Sources:

Photos courtesy of FEMA

This book has drawn heavily on the authoritative materials published by a wide range of sources.

These materials are in the public domain, but accreditation has been given both in the text and in the reference section if you need additional information.

The author and publisher have taken great care in the preparation of this handbook, but make no expressed or implied warranty of any kind and assume no responsibility for errors or omissions.

No liability is assumed for incidental or consequential damages in connection with or arising out of the use of the information or recommendations contained herein.

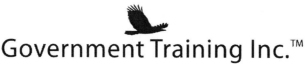

Government Training Inc.™

Physical Security & Grants

For more information on the company, its publications and professional training,
go to http://www.governmenttraininginc.com

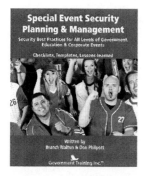

Special Event Security Planning & Management
Security Best Practices for All Levels of Government, Education & Corporate Events

Don Philpott, a recognized international writer on security solutions, and Branch Walton, former U.S. Secret Service and corporate security advisor, have teamed-up to bring to the reader security best practices for events planning. The book draws on national and regional events lessons-learned and "right-sized" planning for all levels of government, education and corporate events. From local parades and public events to major sports and entertainment—all can use this practical guide.

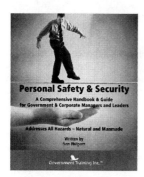

Personal Safety & Security
A Comprehensive Handbook & Guide for Government & Corporate Managers and Leaders

We all have a duty to our families, friends and loved ones to ensure that the places where we live, work, learn and play are secure, and that the people using them are safe.

The aim of this Handbook is not to alarm you, but to prepare and protect you. In the event of a disaster or terrorist incident, first responders may not be able to get to you immediately. Our goal is to give you the information you need so that you are aware of the various threats you face and how to recognize and respond to them.

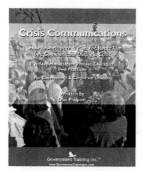

Crisis Communications
How to Anticipate and Plan For, React To, and Communicate During a Crisis

Crisis planning and communications is an integral part of good management practice. By anticipating potential problem areas, identifying solutions, and being prepared you instantly remove a lot of the confusion and anxiety that arise when a crisis does occur.

If people know what to do, they can get on with performing their designated tasks immediately and, as a team, tackle the problem and get back to normal as quickly as possible.

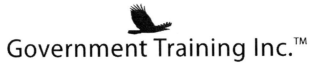

Government Training Inc.™

Physical Security & Grants

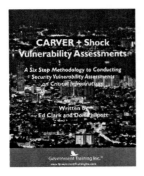

CARVER + Shock Vulnerability Assessment Tool
A 6-Step Approach to Conducting Security Vulnerability Assessments on Critical Infrastructuree

CARVER has served as the standard for security vulnerability assessments for many years. It has now morphed into an even more useful tool that can be used to help protect almost any critical infrastructure.

This new, no-nonsense handbook provides the security professional with background on CARVER, one of its very successful morphs into CARVER + Shock, and then demonstrates how these methodologies can be applied and adapted to meet today's specific needs to protect both hard and soft targets.

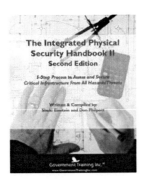

The Integrated Physical Security Handbook II
2nd Edition
5-Step Process to Assess and Secure Critical Infrastructure From All Hazards Threats

This new edition covers a number of additional areas including convergence of systems, building modeling, emergency procedures, privacy issues, cloud computing, shelters and safe areas, and disaster planning. There is also a comprehensive glossary as well as access to a dedicated website at www.physicalsecurityhandbook.com that provides purchasers of the book an online library of over 300 pages of additional reference materials.

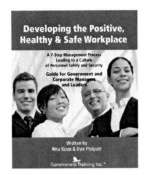

Developing the Positive, Healthy & Safe Workplace
A 7-Step Management Process Leading to a Culture of Personnel Safety & Security

Rita Rizzo is a nationally recognized expert on all aspects of workplace quality, employee development, leadership and workplace security. Her thought-provoking seminars and books have brought practical solutions to the challenges of leadership. In the book, Rita presents a 7-step process for use by management and staff to create a positive, healthy, and safe workplace.

Government Training Inc.™

Physical Security & Grants

For more information on the company, its publications and professional training,
go to http://www.governmenttraininginc.com

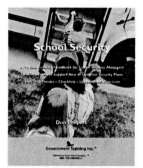

School Security
A Physical Security Handbook for School Security Managers

The School Security Handbook provides an easy to follow and implement 5-step process for developing an emergency response plan that covers almost any eventuality. It covers the phases of an emergency: mitigation and prevention, preparedness, response, and recovery.

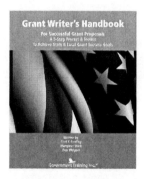

Grant Writer's Handbook
A 5-Step Process & Toolkit to Achieve State & Local Grant Success Goals

The easy to follow 5-step process leads you through the tortuous world of grant writing—starting with how to select the right grant writer, and then following the process from where to find grants to writing winning grant submissions.

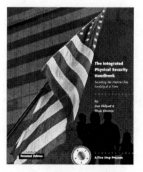

The Integrated Physical Security Handbook
Securing the Nation One Facility at a Time

The Integrated Physical Security Handbook has become the recognized manual for commercial and government building and facility security managers responsible for developing security plans based on estimated risks and threats—natural or terrorist-based.

About the authors

Mary Russell, EdD, MSN

Mary Russell, EdD, MSN works under contract for Florida Department of Health's Bureau of Preparedness and Response's Hospital Preparedness Program as a Hospital Project Manager. Her background includes serving as a prior chairperson and current Steering and General Committee member for the Healthcare Emergency Response Coalition (HERC) for Palm Beach County, FL; as a member of her county's Medical Reserve Corps, and continuing to work night-shift per diem in the Emergency Department of Boca Raton Regional Hospital as an ER nurse.

Her educational background includes a bachelor's degree from Russell Sage College in Troy, NY; a master's in nursing from Pace University in Pleasantville, NY; and a doctorate in education from Florida International University in Miami. She has worked in numerous settings, including critical care, burn units, community health settings, and other areas of practice beyond the emergency department setting. Her background includes involvement in a series of disasters, including the need for emergency evacuation.

James (Jim) Kendig, MS, CHSP, CHCM, HEM, LHRM

Vice President Safety, Security, Clinical/Courier Transportation – Health First

James Kendig is a Vice President and Safety Officer for Health First. He is the Immediate Past President of the Florida Society for Healthcare Security, Safety, & Emergency Management Professionals (a Florida Hospital Association professional membership group). Jim is also a Joint Commission Surveyor specializing in Emergency Management, Environment of Care, and Life Safety. Jim is also the co-chair of the State of Florida's Medical Equipment Committee. Jim is co-chair of the Health First Patient Safety Committee. Jim holds a Bachelor and Master's degree from West Chester University, West Chester, PA. He is a Certified Security Executive (CSE), Certified Healthcare Safety Professional (CHSP), Certified Hazard Control Manager (CHCM), Certified Healthcare Environmental Manager (HEM) through ECRI, and is a former certified OSHA Instructor. Mr. Kendig is a faculty member of the University of Central Florida's Risk Management program and is a Licensed Healthcare Risk Manager (LHRM) in the State of Florida. He has published a number of Environment of Care related articles for Joint Commission's Environment of Care News, the International Association for Healthcare Security and Safety (IAHSS), The Florida Police Chiefs Association, HCPro, FHA, EC News, and other nursing and non-nursing journals and periodicals. He has presented to audiences throughout the country regarding the Environment of Care including the Florida Hospital Association, the Georgia Hospital Association, VHA Southeast, VHA Mid-America, VHA Mountain States, Ohio Hospital Association, New Jersey Hospital Association, IAHSS, Florida Society of Clinical Oncology, Michigan's D1RMRC, and Alabama Society for Healthcare Risk Management and other specialty groups. He is recognized VHA mock surveyor specializing in the Environment of Care. He is a former member of NFPA's Technical Committee on Healthcare Emergency Management as a voting member and has assisted in the publication of HCPro's "Safety Rick Assessment Tools – Strategies for Joint Commission Compliance," ECRI's "Physician Office Fundamentals in Risk Management and Patient Safety," and several chapters in the IAHSS safety and security officers training manual, and ECRI's "Falls Prevention Strategies in Healthcare Settings," among others. Jim has also produced videos on workplace violence and national videos on surge capacity. He is currently part of the EPA's Pharmaceutical Waste Stakeholder Outreach committee and is a board member on ECRI's HEM program. Jim and his team have written the first hospital Pandemic Flu Plan in Florida and the first hospital based Chempack plan as well as the first hospital based POD plan. He also led the state initiative to standardize emergency management codes and participated in the standardization of the state-wide patient wrist-band project, infant and pediatric abduction and abandonment toolkit, forensic patient management toolkit (all available on FHA's web site). Jim and team also developed the first web based hospital evacuation tool for Florida and will be working with VHA agreement hospitals to drill this new tool. Jim is a World Class Leader for Health First and has been awarded dozens of team awards and the organization's Presidents award and Golden Eagle award. Jim is a former law enforcement officer from Pennsylvania.

Don Philpott

Don Philpott is editor of International Homeland Security Journal and has been writing, reporting and broadcasting on international events, trouble spots and major news stories for almost 40 years. For 20 years he was a senior correspondent with Press Association-Reuters, the wire service, and traveled the world on assignments including Northern Ireland, Lebanon, Israel, South Africa and Asia.

He writes for magazines, and newspapers in the United States and Europe, and is a regular contributor to radio and television programs on security and other issues. He is the author of more than 100 books on a wide range of subjects and has had more than 5,000 articles printed in publications around the world. His most recent books are Handbooks for COTRs, Performance Based Contracting, Cost Reimbursable Contracting, How to Manage Teleworkers, Crisis Communications and Integrated Physical Security Handbook II. He is a member of the National Press Club.

Contents

Notice:

Appendices & Blank Forms are available online. To access additional materials, visit our website at www.GovernmentTrainingInc.com, go to the Books section of the website, and click on Physical Security Planning for Medical Facilities. In the Reference Library Login area of the page, use the following credentials to login:

Username: GTI246686

Password: 09119781

This username and password are assigned to you, the purchaser. You will need to enter your email address when logging in so that we can verify each visitor. This information is for the use of the purchaser only and not to be distributed to anyone except the purchaser.

Symbols

Throughout this book you will see a number of icons displayed. The icons are there to help you as you work through the Six Step process. Each icon acts as an advisory – for instance alerting you to things that you must always do or should never do. The icons used are:

 This is something that you must always do

 This is something you should never do

 Really useful tips

 Points to bear in mind

 Have you checked off or answered everything on this list?

Introduction

This book, while focusing on hospitals, is aimed at all health care providers – from the largest hospital to the smallest private nursing home. (Remember)In the event of an emergency, the challenges facing them all are the same even though the logistics are very different. However, they are all part of the emergency planning system and should be prepared for accordingly.

The National Response Framework (NRF), published by the Department of Homeland Security in 2008, serves as a guide for all response agencies at every level in the United States, including hospitals, to use common training, language and responses as an all-hazards approach to disasters. This unified national response to disasters recommends using Incident Command System (ICS) language for response roles and referencing job action sheets for responsibilities associated with those roles.

Hospitals use a Hospital Incident Command System (HICS) approach which is aligned with the National Incident Management System (NIMS) and the way other response agencies are directed to act. This includes local, county, regional, state, tribal and federal levels. Hospitals need to comply with NIMS objectives if they receive federal preparedness and response grants, contracts or cooperative agreement funds.

Two other resources that should be taken into account are the National Security Strategy May 2010 and the National Infrastructure Protection Plan 2009, both of which stress the importance of an integrated, multi-agency approach in emergency planning to protect people and the critical infrastructure they depend on.

While most health care providers, especially hospitals, have emergency plans in place, many smaller health care facilities do not. Hospitals and nursing homes are required to have emergency plans in place to cope with manmade, technological and natural disasters using an "all hazards" approach. The Centers for Medicare & Medicaid Services requires hospitals and nursing homes that receive Medicare or Medicaid payments to maintain and exercise emergency plans.

The Joint Commission (TJC) requires that hospitals and nursing homes it accredits maintain and exercise emergency plans that include processes for evacuations. Hospital and nursing home administrators often have the responsibility for deciding whether to evacuate their patients or to shelter in place during a disaster. State and local governments can order evacuations of the population or segments of the population during emergencies. However, following Hurricanes Rita and Katrina, every effort is likely to be made to evacuate if required.

Hospital administrators usually evacuate only as a last resort, and facilities' emergency plans are designed primarily to shelter in place. Even when county or state officials recommend that hospitals and nursing homes evacuate their facilities, the final decision is made by either the hospital or nursing home administrator.

> Both options – shelter in place and evacuation – must be considered as part of emergency planning.

The facility must have adequate resources to shelter in place. Examples of resources include space, staff, and supplies and power. Without these resources, a facility may be unable to care for patients at the facility, and therefore may be more likely to evacuate.

 Must Do ───────────

This is why it is important to coordinate with county emergency management officials.

Risks to patients must be considered in deciding when to evacuate – for instance, when a hurricane threatens. Evacuating too soon may place patients needlessly at risk if the potential threat does not materialize. Evacuating at the same time as the general public may increase risk to patients' health if traffic congestion and other road complications increase travel time.

Evacuating too late increases risk if patients do not arrive at their destination before a storm strikes.

Evacuating a hospital or nursing home requires a facility to secure transportation to move patients and a receiving facility to accept patients. Facilities are likely to have arrangements for these services locally, but they are less likely to have arrangements with organizations in other localities or states, as was necessary for an event such as Hurricane Katrina. Some states such as Florida, for instance, with a long history of hurricanes, do have such arrangements in place, and hospitals, as one example, use a VHA agreement that allows 32 healthcare systems to reach out during an event. The agreement covers Florida and Alabama. Other examples in Florida include the Disaster Aid Services to Hospitals DASH agreements and the Healthcare Emergency Response Coalition (HERC) of Palm Beach County.

Hospitals and nursing homes accept that their contracted transportation providers may be limited in being able to support them during a major disaster because local demand for transportation will likely exceed supply.

The destruction of facility infrastructure during a storm may force a facility administrator to decide to evacuate after the event, due to building damage or a lack of utilities. For example, a nursing home in Florida evacuated after Hurricane Charley in 2004 because the facility's roof was destroyed and the facility lost power and water service. Many hospitals stop elective surgeries 30-36 hours prior to anticipated hurricane landfall to decrease pre-storm census.

The destruction of community infrastructure, such as the loss of communications systems and transportation routes, can further complicate the decision to evacuate. For example, during Hurricane Katrina, the destruction of communications systems left hospital and nursing home administrators unable to receive basic information such as when assistance would arrive.

Nursing home administrators must also consider additional factors. Nursing home administrators told us that they cannot reduce the number of residents because residents generally have no other home and cannot care for themselves. In contrast, hospital administrators told us that it is common to discharge as many patients as possible before a disaster to reduce the number of patients who need to be sheltered or evacuated and to make room for post storm "casualties."

When a nursing home evacuates, the administrator must locate receiving facilities that can accommodate residents for a potentially long period. For example, a nursing home in Florida had to relocate residents for more than 10 months because of damage to the facility. Despite the problems, all nursing homes need an evacuation plan, and they must practice it.

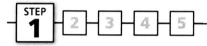

STEP 1
Planning

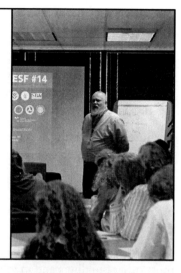

Most Americans are accustomed to receiving sophisticated and prompt medical attention after an injury or when a medical problem presents, anytime and anywhere in the country, without traveling great distances. Such expectations are even greater during mass emergencies that require immediate care for a large number of casualties. In circumstances in which hospital operations are disrupted or completely disabled, the adverse effects of such disasters can be quickly compounded, frequently with catastrophic results. A report from the Congressional Research Service (CRS), Hurricane Katrina: the Public Health and Medical Response examined the performance of the public health system during this devastating event.

According to the CRS report, Hurricane Katrina pushed some of the most critical health care delivery systems to their limits for the first time in recent memory (Lister, 2005).

 Remember ——————

Therefore, the importance of uninterrupted hospital operations and ready access to, and availability of, immediate medical care cannot be exaggerated.

The situation is even more complex when hospitals and other health care facilities have to evacuate patients and staff for whatever reason. In Florida, there are many hospitals close to the coast. While the hospitals may be able to remain operational after a hurricane, the homes of many of the staff may have been destroyed. Your planning has to take this sort of situation into account – does your staff report for duty and you provide accommodation for them or are they released from duty to be with their families and literally pick up the pieces? At Cape Canaveral Hospital, Florida, 85 percent of the staff lives beachside. This could potentially have a big impact for post-storm staffing.

> Different natural and manmade phenomena present different challenges, and each hazard requires a different approach and a different set of actions.

When communities face more than one of these hazards, i.e., they are in an area prone to flooding and tornadoes, the planning team must select the mitigation measures most appropriate for achieving the desired performance level, regardless of the immediate cause for the potential losses.

For instance, flooding is a more site-specific hazard than others. The preferred approach for new facilities is to select a site that is not subject to flooding. When that is not feasible, site modifications or other site-specific building design features that mitigate anticipated flood hazard will reduce the potential for damage. In extreme circumstances, when the hazard becomes so great that the only course of action is to evacuate the facility, plans have to be in place to enable this to happen in an orderly and timely manner while it is still possible.

The orderly evacuation of a hospital is an entirely different process from that recommended for most other buildings and involves special considerations. Due to the fact that so many patients may be medically unstable and dependent on life-support or mechanical equipment, complete evacuation of the facility is to be initiated only as a last resort, and must proceed in a planned and orderly manner. As the NFPA says, "Patients are routinely unable to be self-sufficient."

Events most likely to trigger activation of an emergency, and possibly an evacuation, plan are:

- Severe weather
- Large external accident – commercial plane crash or similar
- Loss of essential utilities including generator
- Large internal accident – contamination, infectious outbreak
- Fire
- Bomb
- Radiation leak or threat of (internal/external)
- Terrorism (chemical, biological attack)

 Must Do

An Evacuation Plan (EP) must be developed and constantly reviewed, updated and practiced.

The plan should be maintained by the appropriate department with the cooperation of all departments within the hospital. Every department within should be responsible for implementing the protocol and for maintaining up-to-date disaster procedures in their work area. Departments should notify the appropriate department at the hospital if significant changes or alterations in their departments transpire which could impact implementation or performance of the plan. The EP should be reviewed at least annually and updated regularly or as major changes/events in the facility occur. The hospital should conduct a scheduled review of the plan and coordinate updates with hospital emergency programs.

The purpose of the EP is to save lives. It is intended to provide for the safety of the staff, patients, visitors and others within the facility during a response to an emergency where partial or full patient evacuation may be required.

When you activate an emergency response or evacuation plan, it has an impact far beyond your facility and can involve hundreds of other people.

Essential staff and patients all have families who are likely to be affected by the same emergency. Key staff cannot function well if they are concerned about loved ones elsewhere. It is important that they have their own personal evacuation plans in place – for themselves and any family pets – as well as essential supplies. The plan should include a predetermined remote destination if there is to be a regional evacuation or a local address – for instance, if mobile home owners are going to a public shelter ahead of a hurricane's landfall. Pets pose a particular problem, as many public shelters do not accept them.

If the emergency calls for essential staff to remain at the facility for an extended period, arrangements should be made in advance for child care, access to cash, emergency support for the employees' homes, PTSD, support for temporary living quarters and so on. The facility's emergency plan might have limited provisions for child care facilities but, depending on the nature of the event, these may not be available at all times.

Overview

Coordination of multiple agencies would most likely lead to Unified Command at the local level with scalability to include multi-agency coordination (MAC). There are five designated tiers: Field, Local, Operational Area, Regional and State. Each level is activated as needed.

- ▸ **Field** – Commands emergency response personnel and resources to carry out tactical decisions and activities in direct response to an incident or threat.

- ▸ **Local** – Manages and coordinates the overall emergency response and recovery activities within their jurisdiction.

- ▸ **Operational Area** – Manages and/or coordinates information, resources and priorities among local governments within the operational area, and serves as the coordination and communication link between the local government level and the regional level.

- ▸ **Regional** – Manages and coordinates information and resources among operational areas within the mutual aid region designated, and between the operational areas and the state level. This level, along with the state level, coordinates overall state agency support for emergency response activities.

- **State** – Manages state resources in response to the emergency needs of the other levels, manages and coordinates mutual aid among the mutual aid regions and between the regional level and state level, and serves as the coordination and communication link with the federal disaster response system.

Additionally, Local Government, Operational Area, Regional and State levels shall provide for all of the following functions within the Standardized Emergency Management System (SEMS):

- **Command Center** – For overall emergency policy and coordination through the joint efforts of governmental agencies and private organizations. Intelligence experts report to the Safety and Security Office within the Command Team.

- **Operations** – For coordinating all jurisdictional operations in support of the response to the emergency through implementation of the organizational level's action plan.

- **Planning** – For collecting, evaluating, and disseminating information; developing the organizational level's action plan in coordination with the other functions; and maintaining documentation.

- **Logistics** – For providing facilities, services, personnel, equipment and materials.

- **Finance** – For financial activities and administrative aspects not assigned to the other functions.

Risk/Vulnerability Assessment

While visitors do not have unrestricted access to most areas of the facility, it is still possible that they may enter departments or clinical areas where they should not be allowed. In addition, hospitals have pharmacies which can be a target for criminals and addicts, they have expensive equipment which can be stolen and, above all, they have patients and visitors who are at their most vulnerable.

 Remember ——————

Hospitals pose particular security challenges because people are coming and going around the clock.

Security is essential to protect both patients and visitors and to control those who would do harm.

To prevent newborn babies from being abducted, strangers should not have access to the pediatrics and obstetrics (mother/baby) units; gifts shops and cafes handling money need to be protected; and sensitive personal health data – both patients and staff – must be safeguarded. Other security issues include hazardous materials onsite, including chemical and radiological, oxygen storage tanks, NO2, and so on.

Some of these security needs are obvious and some are not. In order to determine what needs to be done, you must first conduct a risk assessment to identify all risks. Once you know what risks you face, you can take steps to eliminate or mitigate them.

Some of these risks can be tackled immediately to resolve the problem. The risk assessment might flag inadequate lighting in the visitor parking lot or unprotected utility hatches. These issued can be addressed. Other threats might only arise as a result of a terrorist attack or severe weather. That is why you need a comprehensive emergency plan allowing you to focus on priority issues identified by your operation's "hazard vulnerability analysis."

The plan sets out exactly what must be done in the event of all your identified "what if" scenarios. The plan must cover what should be done and who does it and must cover everything that could possible happen, including a catastrophic event that would force the evacuation of the entire facility.

Hazard Vulnerability Analysis

Hazard Vulnerability Analysis (HVA) is a way to focus attention on those hazards that are most likely to have an impact on your facility and the surrounding community. It is intended that the HVA be seen as an evolving document and be reviewed at least annually. There are four categories that are used to help place each hazard into perspective. These categories are Probability, Response, Human Impact and Property Impact on a facility. Each of these categories is based on a points system, ranging from 0 to 3. For each hazard, a point estimate of 0 (NA) to 3 (high) is given for each of the four categories.

There are many hazards that a hospital may face, but among the most potentially disastrous are bomb threats or terrorist attack; serious fire (requiring assistance from the local fire department and evacuation); floods, tornadoes or other serious thunderstorm activity; winter weather (including blizzards, ice or snow storms, freezing temperatures); and blackouts. Other possible hazards include workplace violence, HVAC failure, water service interruption, phone and Internet failure, medical gas failure and disease/infection outbreak.

> Hospitals have to consider the probability of each hazard occurring and determine the most appropriate response.

Administrators should assess probability based on the known risk, historical information and statistics. Certain hazards are highly unlikely for hospitals in certain areas and should, thereby, be given less of a priority. For instance, a blizzard is an unlikely hazard for a hospital in Miami, but a thunderstorm is a serious and likely threat. Hospital officials must develop the most efficient and cost-effective response that would protect the greatest number of patients.

Hospitals must consider three primary categories of impact for each hazard: the human impact, property impact and business impact. Human impact, which is of course most important, is the measure of potential staff and patient deaths and injuries. Property impact encompasses time and cost to replace or repair infrastructure, and the time and cost to provide temporary solutions. Business impact includes many areas, but mainly the effects on workers, administrators, suppliers, future patients, legal costs and future reputation. The administrators must analyze the hazards, probability and impacts all together.

An example of an HVA can be seen at www.njha.com/ep/pdf/627200834041PM.pdf.

Risk Mitigation

The first step must be to try to mitigate the impact of risks or hazards.

> A full evacuation should only be considered as a last resort.

In order to develop evacuation strategies, facilities should first inspect their surrounding environments for hazards that pose further risks to evacuees and facility operations. Attention should be given to the various elements of evaluation.

Potential Vulnerabilities

Hospitals usually have high levels of occupancy, with patients, staff and many visitors present 24 hours a day. Visitors are not just those people visiting a patient and restricted to hospital visiting hours. They include vendors, students, faith community members, consultants and contractors.

Many patients require constant attention, and in many cases continuous and specialized care, and the use of sophisticated medical instruments or other equipment. Hospital operations also depend on a steady supply of medical and other types of material, as well as public services or lifelines. In addition, hospital vulnerability is aggravated by the presence of hazardous substances that may be spilled or released in a hazard event.

Given the importance of hospital services for response and recovery following emergencies, and the need for uninterrupted operation of these facilities, hospital administrators and designers must consider all aspects of their vulnerability. Three main aspects of hospital vulnerability must be taken into account:

- Structural
- Nonstructural
- Organizational

Structural Vulnerability

Structural vulnerability is related to potential damage to structural components of a building. They include foundations, weight-bearing walls, columns and beams, staircases, floors and roof decks, or other types of structural components that help support the building. The level of vulnerability of these components depends on the following factors:

- The level to which the design of the structural system has addressed the hazard forces
- The quality of building materials, construction and maintenance
- The architectural and structural form or configuration of a building

Buildings may be vulnerable from wind, flooding, earthquakes and wildfires. The aspects of adequate design and construction in most hazard-prone areas are regulated by building codes and other regulations, i.e., southeastern hospitals are built to withstand hurricane-force winds while facilities in the southwest have to be able to withstand earthquakes and those in the midwest are in the tornado belt.

The main purpose of these regulations is to protect the safety of occupants. They are usually prescriptive in nature, i.e., they establish minimum requirements that are occasionally updated based on newly acquired knowledge.

 Remember ———————————

Because of the threat of terrorism, hospitals also have to be protected from explosive devices which can cause structural collapse and serious injury from flying glass and other debris.

Once you have established the structural threats you can take steps to mitigate the risks, i.e., installing impact glass in exterior windows, hardening doors and even adding additional columns to reinforce weight-bearing walls. The building regulations alone, however, cannot guarantee uninterrupted operation of a hospital, because a great many other factors affect hospital functions.

Other important areas to be considered when reviewing structural vulnerability are safe areas and shelter-in-place locations. Most hospitals prefer to shelter in place rather than evacuate – unless the situation is so critical they have to – but they may not have undertaken an assessment of how they could quickly bring patients and staff to "safe" areas in their facilities in the event of an emergency such as a tornado.

Nonstructural Vulnerability

The experience of hospital evacuations and other types of disruption during recent hazard events (many of which are described in greater detail in later chapters) has heightened the awareness that hospital functions could be seriously impaired or interrupted, even when the facilities did not sustain significant structural damage. The effects of damage to nonstructural building components and equipment, as well as the effects of breakdowns in public services (lifelines), transportation, resupply or other organizational aspects of hospital operations can be as disruptive, and as dangerous for the safety of patients, as any structural damage.

Nonstructural vulnerabilities that can affect hospital functions and the safety of occupants include the potential failures of architectural components, both on the exterior and the interior of buildings.

Damage to roof coverings, facades or windows can make way for water penetration that can damage sensitive equipment and shut down many hospital functions. When roofing material is disturbed by wind, the roof may start to leak and the moisture can knock out vital equipment, disrupt patient care, and penetrate walls and other concealed spaces, allowing mold to build up over time. An example is when hospitals in South Florida went through a series of hurricanes within a few weeks in 2004 and many facilities experienced water leaks. This was noted after ceiling tiles started falling down, burdened down by water. It became a hazard for staff in hallways and for patients in their rooms.

Window breakage resulting from high winds, earthquakes and even flooding frequently requires patient evacuation from affected areas. A sprinkler pipe break can cause flooding that requires some temporary relocation. Patients in critical care and acute care units are particularly vulnerable because the move separates them from medical gas outlets, monitors, lighting and other essential support services.

Non-weight-bearing and partition walls and ceilings, for instance, are rarely designed and constructed to the same standards of hazard resistance as the structural elements. Collapse of these components has caused a number of evacuations and closures of hospitals following a hazard event.

Other nonstructural vulnerabilities that must be considered include:

- Communication equipment that supports internal and external transmissions
- Protections against cyber-terrorism
- Safeguards and redundancy for utilities (power, water, fuel, etc.)
- Oxygen storage areas
- Deliveries of radioisotopes

Installations

Hospitals are extremely complex building systems that depend on an extensive network of mechanical, electrical and piping installations. The air and ventilation system is one of the most important because it is responsible for maintaining an appropriate environment in different parts of the hospital. Isolation rooms may be equipped with negative pressure airflow so that harmful airborne organisms do not migrate outside the patient's room and infect others.

Plan on isolation-cohorting of patients in the event of a biologic outbreak affecting a lot of patients or consider building modifications to allow for providing for negative pressure in large areas of the hospital.

There are not a lot of Airborne Infection Isolation Rooms (AIIRS), and hospitals should consider planning to convert an entire unit or even a tent alternative care site with negative pressure in the event of an emergency.

Floors or units housing patients with immune system deficiencies require a positive pressure differential, so that harmful organisms do not enter the patients' rooms and needlessly infect them. The malfunction in any one part of this ventilation system could create a risk of infection to patients and staff. This system is extremely vulnerable to disruption as a result of indirect building damage. Winds can overturn improperly attached roof-mounted ventilation and air-conditioning equipment, while the ductwork is very susceptible to collapse in earthquakes. Additionally, strong winds may change the airflow from ventilation exhaust outlets, potentially causing harmful discharges from patient care areas and the clinical laboratory to be sucked back into the fresh air intakes. Airborne debris from windstorms could quickly clog the air filtration systems, making them inoperable or impaired.

Hospitals depend on several essential piping systems. Medical gases are among the most important, along with water, steam and fire sprinkler systems. Physicians and nurses depend on oxygen and other gasses and suction required for patient care. Unless properly secured and braced, these installations can be easily dislodged or broken, causing dangerous leakage and potential additional damage.

In floods and earthquakes particularly, sewers are apt to overflow, back up or break down. Waste disposal is essential for any hospital, because when the toilets back up, or sterilizers, dishwashers, and other automated cleaning equipment cannot be discharged and water is no longer available for dialysis patients, patient care is immediately affected. Retention ponds or holding tanks coupled with backflow and diversion valves can be employed to solve this problem; however, in many hospitals, this issue has not been adequately addressed.

 Must Do

The emergency power supply system is probably the most critical element in this group. Together with fuel supply and storage facilities, this system enables all the other hospital installations and equipment that have not sustained direct physical damage to function normally in any disaster. So it is important to plan where your generator and other essential components of your electrical distribution system are located.

Elevator service is vulnerable not only to power outages, but also to direct damage to elevator installations. Water penetration also damages the elevator sensors that impact the controls. Mitigation through the installation of louvers limits water entry during horizontal-blowing rain conditions. Usually only one or two elevators are placed on the emergency power system. Without functioning elevators, vertical patient evacuation or staff transport to upper or lower floors of a hospital become difficult exercises.

In the event of an earthquake, elevator shafts and other equipment can be damaged or dislodged, effectively shutting down the building. Flooding of elevator pits was a common problem during Hurricane Katrina and was responsible for the loss of elevator service.

However, uninterrupted operation of a hospital during a power outage is possible only if adequate electrical wiring is installed in all the areas that require uninterrupted power supply. Since extra wiring and additional circuits for emergency power increase the initial construction costs of the building, the decision on the emergency power coverage requires a thorough evaluation of the relative vulnerability of various functions to power outage. As patients become more critically ill and the nature of diagnosis and treatment becomes more dependent on computers, monitors and other electrical equipment, the need for emergency power will continue to grow.

When the series of four hurricanes hit Florida in 2004, patients were evacuated into the hallways to protect them from the potential threat of window breakage from the high winds and tornadoes. These days, patients are connected to all sorts of electrical equipment, including intravenous pumps, analgesic delivery devices, nasogastric suction, chest tubes, antithrombotic devices and others, making it difficult to move them out of their room.

The experience of Hurricane Katrina has demonstrated the need for emergency power coverage even for services that typically have not been regarded as critical, such as climate control and air-conditioning systems. Extreme heat caused a number of hospitals to evacuate their patients and staff when the conditions became unbearable. Climate control can become a patient safety threat and can lead to a need for evacuation if environmental temperatures get too high. Specific laboratory and radiology equipment will also be affected without climate control measures in place.

With hurricanes, big trees overturn and break water main lines, disrupting water supplies and causing lack of water pressure and sewer functioning. Water disruption can interrupt dialysis services, surgical services and be an infection control threat if staff cannot wash their hands frequently.

There are many types of internal hazards that might occur as a result of a disaster. In the past, bottles in clinical laboratories have fallen and started fires. Earthquakes have catapulted filing cabinet drawers and ventilators across rooms at high speed, with the potential of causing considerable injury to personnel. Any wheeled equipment is vulnerable to displacement and has the potential to cause injury.

Hospitals use and depend on many types of communication systems. For communications with emergency vehicles or first-response agencies, hospitals often depend on radio antennas that are frequently mounted on roofs and exposed to high winds and windborne debris impact, even though the base stations are maintained inside the buildings. In Florida, they are placed near roof areas in protected rooms. Satellite dishes, communication masts, antennae and other equipment can be blown off the roof or be severely damaged, leaving the hospital without this vital service at a critical time.

Organizational

Most hospitals have disaster mitigation or emergency operation plans, but not all of them provide organizational alternatives in the event of disruption of the normal movement of staff, patients, equipment and supplies that characterizes everyday hospital operations.

> Hospitals that receive federal funding must be in compliance with the National Incident Management System (NIMS) as part of the National Response Framework (NRF).

Using a Hospital Incident Command approach is associated with a preplanned organizational structure to be able to manage any kind of incident.

The critical nature and interdependence of these processes represent a separate category of vulnerabilities that need careful attention. Spatial distribution of hospital functions and their inter-relationship determines the extent to which hospital operations are affected when normal movement and communication of people, materials and waste are disrupted. The disruption by natural hazard events of administrative services, such as contracting, procurement, maintenance and allocation of resources, can impair hospital functions almost as much as any physical damage.

Just-in-time delivery: Many hospitals have currently eliminated, or greatly reduced, onsite storage for linen, supplies, food and other materials essential to normal operations. Any prolonged isolation or blockage of streets serving the hospital could lead to a need to ration supplies and triage patients for treatment. During Hurricane Katrina, many hospitals were isolated by floodwaters for five or more days and, in many cases, could not replenish critical supplies. In some instances, this contributed to the decision to evacuate the facility. During the H1N1 outbreak, many hospitals faced a shortage of N95 masks (for more information on Evacuation see Step Three).

Risk Assessment and Analysis

There are many methods for identifying, evaluating and defining hazards that may affect a facility. Depending on facility location and size, hazards may require considerable expertise to identify properly. Hazards are not limited to natural events. Technological risks can result in the loss of utilities, information technology or communications equipment. Hazard vulnerability analysis can be provided by knowledgeable staff, software programs, and guidance from local emergency response partners (fire-rescue, law enforcement) and county government emergency planners and consultants. In some states, it is now required that local EM personnel are included in your EM evaluation.

An additional tool in assessment is the use of "lessons learned" from similar incidents. Events that led to evacuation or shelter-in-place decisions can be pinpointed through data from associations, insurance companies, hospital association and community emergency planners/responders. By evaluating information from sources, such as these, facilities are more likely to identify potential hazards.

Frequency

To effectively identify the most likely evacuation scenarios, facilities must first qualify hazards and how often they occur. Frequency is not a stand-alone indicator, since a least-likely scenario may have the largest impact.

Duration of Incident

Each evacuation plan should consider how long a hazard would impact facility operations. An example is a hospital that has sustained such significant structural damage that clinical services cannot continue until major repairs have been made.

Scope of Impact

Plans for evacuation will depend upon how much of the facility is affected, for how long and to what degree.

Destructive Potential to Life and Property

To understand the type and length of evacuation, facility planners should know how much destruction is likely from the risk at hand. If a flood lasts for three weeks and covers the entire structure, patients may be transferred for months to other sites. A chemical release or a patient presenting with chemical contamination, however, may have little destructive impact on the facility structure, but result in risk to patients and staff and restricted services until contaminants are contained and removed.

Controllability

Facility planners cannot control all hazards but may be able to reduce vulnerabilities through mitigation interventions and planning.

Predictability

Based on past history, some events may be predictable. The ability to reasonably predict events will assist in planning for evacuation. An example would include the building and grounds being routinely flooded during high-rainfall years.

Speed of Onset

Every facility should have a method to quickly identify events that will create an immediate threat.

In some cases, staff may have many days for planning and decision-making or have very little time to react. Lack of time to prepare can have a substantial impact on the health of patients and staff. Facility planners should find methods to provide early warning to staff for those events that can require evacuations within minutes of occurrence (e.g. earthquake, fire, tornado, levee break, etc.)

Length of Forewarning

> The longer delays occur in response to a disaster, the fewer options are available to react successfully.

Equipping facilities with appropriate warning systems will maximize the response time for evacuation or sheltering decisions. These may include weather radios that activate immediately upon a warning from the National Weather Service, an automated warning service provided by phone, or a warning siren from a nuclear power plant. Facility staff should also be trained to identify local sirens or messages provided on radio or television by the Emergency Alert System or other internal mechanisms. In hospitals, the use of overhead announcements and mass notification systems are critical.

Developing Facility Protective Actions

There are several strategies for evacuation which include:

- Sheltering in place without moving clients
- Sheltering in place to a safe area on the same level (horizontal relocation)
- Sheltering in place vertically (up or down)
- Evacuating just outside the facility
- Evacuating to a nearby like facility
- Evacuating to a distant like facility
- Evacuating to a shelter designated as a medical treatment unit (and originating facility continues to provide all staff and support services)
- Evacuating to a shelter designated as a medical treatment unit (and local health officials provide all staff and support services)
- Evacuating to a general public shelter with a temporary infirmary

NOTE: When considering movement of patients, whether within or outside the facility, facility planners must consider the inherent risk that the travel will impact the individual's health, particularly with critical care patients of any age.

Sheltering in place without moving clients

Depending on the degree of risk, facility staff may decide to remain in place because the threat may have less impact on client health and safety than a voluntary evacuation.

- **Example:** A facility becomes aware of an external community chemical release that will affect it within a short period of time, and local government advises staying indoors or evacuating the area. Evacuation could expose patients/residents to greater risks than sheltering in place; however, action must be taken to address the HVAC system to minimize contamination entering the building.

Sheltering in place to a safe area or refuge on the same level

An evacuation may be necessary from one side of a building to another, based on an approaching threat.

- **Example:** Staff would be expected to identify the path, speed and appropriate destination of the threat to ensure a timely movement of patients and critical equipment. This is the most preferred option.

Sheltering in place vertically (up or down)

For fast-moving, short-duration events, it may be necessary to move patients above or below their designated floors. This is usually done because time in which to respond to a serious hazard is extremely limited. Lower-level sheltering may be required for high-wind scenarios or during threats from some manmade threat (e.g., a nearby impending explosion). Upper-level sheltering may be required for scenarios involving very fast-moving waters or during the release of ground-hugging chemicals in the immediate area.

▸ **Example:** A two-story facility has a fall-out shelter in the basement. The National Weather Service has announced a tornado warning in the area. A staff member's relative has already seen a funnel cloud touch down less than a mile from the facility. Staff should consider moving patients from the upper floor and those near windows, to the security of the basement or to the core of the building until the tornado warning has subsided. Fire doors work well for containment of multiple hazards, including as a security feature. For example, they can afford an initial layer of protection from a violent person with a weapon.

Evacuating just outside the facility

There may be an internal emergency, which will require staff to evacuate patients from the building. This could be for an immediate problem or a long-duration event. The evacuation plan should include locations where facility staff can perform an inventory of those who have left the building. The plan should also include contingencies for this occurring during inclement weather, and the possible need for further evacuation to nearby like facilities. You should also identify internal locations to support patient care temporarily and to address any influx of patients.

▸ **Example:** Staff of a nursing home smell smoke in the facility and calls 911. They are directed to move patients out of the building. Upon authorization from the fire department, they return indoors.

Evacuating to a nearby like facility

Facilities with medically fragile residents should consider movement of patients/residents and staff to a nearby facility, with like capacity for care of patients/residents. This evacuation type might be considered during a voluntary or precautionary evacuation, and would definitely be appropriate during a mandatory evacuation order. It is critical that facilities have agreements with nearby like facilities to take clients. More than one facility should be identified, usually in opposite directions from the affected facility, in case the primary site is impacted by the same threat. Facilities should identify whether other medical and residential care facilities are also planning to use the same location to receive clients. In addition, plans should address accessible evacuation routes (depending on risks) and transportation assets and logistics.

▸ **Example:** Local government authorities have warned a facility that flood controls may fail within six hours. The facility has a high risk of being flooded within the next two days. Staff have been given adequate time to secure bed space and care, as available, at one or more pre-designated similar level of care facilities. They have also been given time to arrange for transportation and verify a safe route for evacuation.

Evacuating to a distant like facility

Very serious conditions may require a facility to move all patients to a distant site. This can occur during regional events with massive impacts. Examples include events such as widespread flooding, earthquake and civil unrest. This choice would be preferable to movement to a nearby medical shelter if the impact of the event will have a substantial duration (more than three or four days) and/or there are extensive equipment and personnel support needs for the care of the patients.

During emergency evacuation, hospitals will transfer their patients to a facility with a similar level of care. Transfer agreements can extend beyond the immediate surrounding geographic area to include further in-state or even out-of-state facilities. Those hospitals located in vulnerable areas at risk of a catastrophic event should plan for such an extreme scenario in which local health infrastructure has been severely damaged and can no longer sustain services.

▸ **Example:** A large earthquake has severely damaged a facility, and staff determines that other local facilities providing the same level of care with which they have agreements, are also disabled and unable to receive additional patients.

Evacuating to a shelter designated as a medical treatment unit (and originating facility continues to provide all staff and support services).

A rapid onset of a disaster may severely limit evacuation and transfer options available to the local emergency authorities and facility. Under these conditions, the local disaster authority may instruct a facility to evacuate and transfer the entire operation to a pre-determined temporary shelter (i.e., school gymnasium) and continue to provide all care and treatment. This option is desirable for short-term evacuations. However, depending on the duration of the event, this may be the first step before transferring patients to another like facility in another geographic area unaffected by the disaster. One issue, however, is if the patient needs med gasses and they are not available.

▸ **Example:** A nearby river is at flood stage and threatens to break through containment levees. If this occurs, the nearby facility will be flooded. A lawful evacuation order has been issued, and the facility has been directed to move all patients and staff to a school gymnasium on higher ground. Patients, staff, equipment and supplies must be transferred with the patients, and the facility must be capable of maintaining operations for a minimum of 96 hours.

Evacuating to a shelter designated as a medical treatment unit (and local health officials provide all staff and support services).

When the scope of the disaster conditions are severe, facility planners may need to consider moving patients to a medical shelter before they can be moved to like facilities. Since they will have to be moved twice, this choice can create increased stress on patients, and the quality of care in the shelters may not be equal to the care available to them in the facility from which they are evacuating. This is the planned degradation of care. Depending on the nature of the disaster, there may be other rules and regulations that have to be followed. For instance, in the event of contamination, the EVA requires decontamination first before the collection of effluent or other harmful matter.

▸ **Example:** An urban firestorm has burned down the neighborhood where a facility was located. Staff members were able to evacuate all patients to a local community shelter for the medically fragile, but it has limited capabilities. Facility planners must arrange for movement of patients to a city that is in another county, as soon as the roads are passable and the fire threat is controlled.

Evacuating to a general public shelter with a temporary infirmary

In worst-case scenarios, facilities may have little choice but to evacuate to the nearest available general population shelter. This decision is made only when there is no other option available, and when there is an immediate peril to life and safety of clients if they are not immediately moved to the closest available shelter. The plan must recognize this as a temporary condition requiring immediate triage activities, in coordination with local government, to move the arriving patients to the closest like facility available, whether or not any previous agreements exist.

▸ **Example:** A massive earthquake has rendered a facility unsafe for occupation. Staff members have used every method available to safely move the patients out of the building. The only available shelter is a school auditorium two miles away. There is a temporary infirmary as part of the general population shelter, with limited nursing staff, medical supplies and support. Facility staff will need to set up a working relationship with local government as soon as possible to arrange for the movement of the patients to a like facility.

Facility Vulnerabilities

Mission critical facilities shall include all of the following:

▸ Acute Care
▸ Ambulatory Care
▸ Animal Facility
▸ Boiler Plant
▸ Communications Center
▸ Domiciliary
▸ Drug/Alcohol Rehabilitation
▸ Emergency Command Center
▸ Emergency Generator
▸ Fire/Police Station
▸ Hazardous Material Storage
▸ Hospital
▸ Information Technology
▸ Long-Term Care
▸ Medical Equipment Storage

- Medical Gas Storage
- Medical Records (depending on the status implementing EMR)
- Medical Research
- Mental Health – Inpatient
- Psychiatric Care Facility
- Rehabilitation Medicine
- Security and Law Enforcement
- Water Tower
- Utility Supply Storage Structure
- Fuel Storage Tanks, Oxygen Storage Areas

Security

During an emergency, security has multiple roles to serve including monitoring the facility, equipment and drugs, ensuring the safety of patients, staff and visitors, and providing crowd control.

> Emergency planning must include detailed security responses to cover all eventualities.

If there is an outbreak of a highly contagious virus or multiple casualties from a terrorist bomb, the facility could quickly become inundated with people seeking treatment. Local law enforcement is likely to be stretched to the limit, so the responsibility will fall on facility security to carry out this function. During any emergency the following measures should be taken:

- Lock all non-essential entrances.
- Station security personnel at all entrances (Emergency Department, Hospital Front, Clinic Front, Atrium Circle, Garage Lobby, Purchasing and Dietary Loading Docks, etc.)or delegate this to others.
- Allow access for authorized persons after ID badges have been screened.
- Assist law enforcement and emergency response agencies. Hospitals frequently have to respond to a major incident outside their area which does impact the jurisdiction in which they operate.
- Secure primary treatment areas for authorized personnel only.
- Maintain after-hours key control of elevator operation.
- Monitor and disseminate flow of information from outside sources (i.e., National Weather Service, Emergency Management and State Department of Health). This function will be shared with the Hospital Liaison Officer in the Command Center during a disaster event.

▸ Control vehicular and pedestrian traffic.

▸ Control access to emergency care.

It may be necessary to restrict or close access to parking garages, and if restricted only authorized key personnel with parking passes should be allowed entry. Crowd control may be necessary both within the facility, in ER for instance, and outside. The emergency plan must cover procedures to be put in place if crowd control is necessary and to ensure that the necessary equipment is available to do this – ropes, barriers, etc.

Physical Security

The physical security of facilities requires the use of concentric levels of control and protection to provide progressively enhanced levels of security.

▸ The first point of control should be at the perimeter of the property consisting of fences and other barriers with one or two points of entry through gates controlled by police or other guard personnel. In certain urban sites, the building perimeter may be on the property line. Increased levels of screening of persons and vehicles, as the Department of Homeland Security Threat Levels are changed, must be accommodated at the perimeter without burdening surrounding roads with vehicles waiting to enter the site.

▸ The second point of control should be at the building perimeter consisting of doors and other openings protected as appropriate to the level of protection needed with or without the first point of control. This includes access control hardware, intrusion detection, surveillance, and, at selected entrances at various times, personnel for control and screening.

▸ The third point of control should be to segregate with barriers and hardware generally accessible public and patient areas from staff-only areas such as pharmacy preparation, food preparation, sterile corridors, research laboratories, and building operations and maintenance areas.

▸ The fourth point of control should be to segregate authorized from unauthorized staff areas with barriers and access controls such as card reader-activated hardware. Unauthorized areas may include patient records, laboratories and cash-handling tellers.

▸ The fifth point of control should be to restrict access to restricted areas to a minimum with card-reader access controls, CCTV monitors, intrusion detection alarms, and forced-entry-resistant construction. Restricted access areas may include select agent storage, narcotics storage and pharmaceutical caches, laboratories and COOP sites.

The more effective the perimeter barrier and screening are the less protection is needed within the site, such as between buildings, from patient and visitor parking and the building lobby, and from the site entrance to the other buildings on the site. In highly urban areas where the building may front on a city street with no stand-off or separation, the building and its occupants can only be protected from hazards of breaking and entering, vandalism, and even explosive or armed attack by hardening the building itself to resist, which may lead to undesirable solutions such as façades with minimum openings and a fortress-like appearance.

Crime Prevention Through Environmental Design (CPTED)

CPTED promotes the principles that proper design and effective use of the built environment can lead to a reduction in the fear and incidence of crime and acts of terrorism. CPTED should be used to evaluate site and building designs to create and enhance the concentric circles or layers of security protection.

Security Operation Requirements

Design decisions for the physical security of a mission critical facility should be based on the concentric levels of control and protection – both physical and operational. It is not possible to eliminate all risk to a facility, and every project will face resource limitations. Cost-effective risk management is a requirement of every project. Prior to design development of a new mission critical facility, or major alterations of an existing mission critical facility, a risk assessment must be performed. Cost-effective strategies must be implemented to make the facility capable of mission critical operation.

The first task is to identify the assets and people that need to be protected. Next, a threat assessment is performed to identify and define the threats and hazards that could cause harm to a building and its occupants. After threats and assets are identified, a vulnerability assessment is performed to identify weaknesses. Using the results of the asset, threat and vulnerability assessment, risk can be determined.

Comprehensive protection against the full range of possible natural and manmade threats to facilities would be cost prohibitive, but an appropriate level of protection obtained through the use of these standards can provide for continued operation of mission critical facilities at a reasonable cost.

Site Considerations

The following guidelines could apply to any large hospital facility or campus.

Stand-Off Distance

No vehicle shall be parked or be permitted to travel closer than 50 feet to any mission critical facility.

Perimeter Fences

Perimeter barriers shall consist of fences, walls, a combination of these and gates, as needed for access. The barrier shall be designed to resist forced or surreptitious entry using hand tools, such as by spreading bars of a fence to provide a passable opening. Fences shall have sufficient lateral support to resist overturning by manual force.

Location

The perimeter barrier shall be on or in close proximity to the perimeter of the property.

Height

The perimeter barrier shall have at least eight (8) feet between potential horizontal footholds or be designed with other anti-climb measures.

Material

Fences shall be metal and of heavy industrial-grade construction with bar spacing. Chain link fences and gates shall not be used. Walls shall be reinforced masonry or concrete.

Gates

Gates shall be of the same or similar design and materials as the adjacent fences. Gates shall be access-card operated from the outside or as prescribed by the project manager.

▸ **Pedestrian gates:** Pedestrian and bicycle gates shall swing in the outward direction and shall be fully accessible in width and operation to persons with disabilities.

▸ **Vehicular gates:** Vehicular security gates shall be sliding or cantilevered (no tracks) and only wide enough to accommodate one vehicle lane.

Vehicle and Pedestrian Screening

Security/Guard Gatehouse

Pedestrian and vehicle perimeter entrances shall be provided with enclosed gatehouses for personnel, gate operation, vehicle inspection and information. Gatehouse design shall be compatible with the facility architecture and the neighborhood. Gatehouses shall be heated, air conditioned and lighted to provide an appropriate work environment. Gatehouses shall be provided with power, telephone, intercom, data and other equipment as directed by security/police.

Vehicle Screening Area

Provide adequate space to accommodate vehicle screening without blocking public rights-of-way. The screening area shall provide adequate space and site utilities to accomplish the following tasks:

▸ Visual identity check of driver's license

▸ Visual inspection of vehicle interior, including luggage compartment

▸ Trace element swipes and sensors (for high-security facilities)

Stacking space: Stacking space shall be provided for vehicles awaiting inspection outside site entrance and off public roads.

▸ At entrances for employee vehicles, the stacking space shall be sufficient to handle the throughput of vehicles at peak inbound levels.

▸ At public entrances, stacking space shall be sufficient for average visitor vehicle traffic volume and include space to pull a vehicle aside out of the lane of inbound traffic.

Separation: In-bound and out-bound vehicles shall have separate lanes and gates at all vehicular entrances.

Reject lane: A turn-around lane shall be provided on the exterior of the entrance gate to permit vehicles to be sent away without interfering with traffic.

Parking: Parking for two police vehicles shall be provided inside the entrance gate.

Public transportation: Where public transportation is allowed onsite for employees and visitors, space shall be provided for the vehicle to be inspected.

Vehicle Barriers

Active or passive vehicle barriers shall be selected on the appropriateness of the architecture of the facility and the specifics of the site and natural environment.

Active Barriers

Types of active barriers shall be hydraulic wedges or bollards recessed into the pavement for a flush condition when not deployed.

Locations: Active vehicle barriers shall be located inside all vehicular perimeter entrance and exit gates at a distance that permits guard personnel adequate response time for deployment.

Stationary (Passive) Barriers

Natural or manmade stationary barriers may be used.

▸ Landscaping examples include berms, gullies, boulders, trees and other terrain.

▸ Hardscaping examples include benches and planters.

▸ Structural examples include walls, bollards and cables.

Locations: Adjacent to vulnerable perimeter fences, protection for site utility equipment, at building entrance, and other areas requiring additional protection from vehicles.

Handicapped accessibility: Passive barriers, such as bollards, when placed adjacent to or across a path of pedestrian travel, shall have four (4) feet clear space in between.

Parking

Location

Surface parking: Passenger vehicles shall not be parked or permitted to travel closer than 50 feet to any facility.

Parking structures

Separate from facility: No parking structure, whether onsite or offsite, shall be constructed closer than the following to any facility.

▸ Underground: no limit

▸ Above ground: same as for surface parking

In or under high-security facility, i.e. VA hospital: Parking in or under a facility shall be restricted.

▸ No unscreened visitor vehicle shall be permitted within or under any facility.

▸   Official government-owned vehicles, regularly garaged in the facility and inspected for covertly placed explosives after leaving and returning to the facility, shall be permitted within or under any facility.

▸   At the discretion of security, selected employee-owned vehicles, regularly inspected for covertly placed explosives after leaving and returning to the facility, may be permitted within or under any facility.

Access

From vehicle entrance: Access roads for all vehicles shall allow for separate driveways to the building entrance, service yard or parking.

▸   Separate entrances to the site shall be provided for patients and visitors, employees and staff, emergency, and service and delivery vehicles.

▸   Access roads from entrances to parking for each vehicle type shall be separated, but may be connected for maintenance and emergency vehicles through gates controlled by access cards.

▸   Access roads shall be configured to prevent vehicles from attaining speeds in excess of 25 mph.

▸   Straight-line vehicular approaches to a facility shall be avoided.

Patients and visitors: Parking and access for patients, visitors, and the persons transporting them to and from the facility shall be as convenient as possible to the main entrance, subject to the aforementioned security requirements.

Parking and facility access shall comply with American Disabilities Act (ADA) accessibility requirements. For more information, go to www.ada.gov/2010ADAstandards_index.htm.

▸   Where vehicles are unscreened, make site provisions to accommodate a shuttle service for persons needing assistance.

▸   Provide accessible shuttle stops or shelters in parking areas.

▸   Provide shuttle parking at building entrance.

Emergency: Emergency entrance shall be provided with a small parking area for emergency patients and space for ambulances. Ambulances shall be permitted to approach the building directly and not be subjected to the distance requirements previously mentioned. Consider methods to summon assistance – a call box at the ambulance and ambulatory entrance?

Childcare parents and staff: All requirements for maintaining stand-off distance between vehicles and the building shall apply. Child drop-off and pick-up shall be visible from the office of the childcare/development center and shall be monitored by CCTV. All vehicular areas, onsite and adjacent offsite, including parking and access roads, shall be separated from playground areas by fences designed to prevent children from entering the vehicular areas and vehicles from entering the playground.

Vendors: The stand-off distance and screening requirements previously mentioned should apply. Vendors shall use the delivery vehicle entrance and service yard at the loading dock. Parking shall be provided for vendors in the service yard.

Employees: Where employees share access with patients and visitors, the entrance to the employee parking shall be controlled by a card-actuated gate. Employee parking areas shall be monitored by CCTV. Emergency alert systems, such as blue phones, shall be provided at the discretion of security/police.

> In all of your planning, always remember ADA requirements.

Site Lighting

General Requirements

Provide minimum maintained illumination levels for pedestrian pathways, bicycle and vehicle routes, parking structures, parking lots, wayfinding, signage, pedestrian entrances, and building services which will provide safety and security for personnel, buildings and site.

Lighting shall provide for safety and security without compromising the quality of the site, the environment (including neighboring properties), or the architectural character of the buildings.

Aesthetics: The site lighting shall provide desired illumination and enhancement of trees, landscaping, and buildings without providing dark shadowy areas compromising safety and security.

CCTV: Site lighting shall provide CCTV and other surveillance support with illumination levels and color that assists in proper identification. Lighting shall be coordinated with CCTV cameras to enhance surveillance and prevent interference. Avoid "blinding" CCTV cameras in the placement and selection of fixtures and their "cutoff" angles.

Luminance levels: Illumination levels shall be in compliance with the Illumination Engineering Society of North America (IESNA), and local and state governing agencies.

Signage and wayfinding: Shall be enhanced by site lighting, including providing improved security by assisting pedestrians and vehicles to locate their destinations expeditiously.

Environmental: Minimize light pollution and spill into neighboring properties by selection of fixtures' cutoff angles to minimize their nuisance visibility from adjacent areas on and off property.

Lighting Locations

Comply with all local/state requirements for site lighting. The following areas require additional attention in lighting design to support security and safety needs.

Site entrances: Lighting shall be provided at all site entrances at illumination levels that assist in after-dark performance of security duties –

▸ To assist security with visual personal identification into vehicles to see the driver's compartment and view ID.

▸ To provide illumination of wayfinding and other signage.

▸ Perimeter fence: Lighting sufficient to support perimeter CCTV surveillance shall be provided without objectionable spill onto neighboring properties or rights-of-way.

▸ Where a perimeter road has been provided for patrols or other functions, the lighting may be combined with roadway lighting.

Building entrances and exits: Lighting at building entrances shall support CCTV surveillance and ID functions while providing illumination of surfaces and features for safety.

Parking areas: All parking areas covered and open shall be lighted in support of CCTV and other surveillance without objectionable spill into adjacent areas onsite or offsite.

Pathways: Pedestrian and bicycle pathways and walks, including bike racks, gates and other features shall be illuminated in support of CCTV and other surveillance while providing for safety without objectionable spill onto adjacent areas onsite and offsite.

Signage: All signage shall be adequately illuminated to provide safe wayfinding and identification. Wayfinding maps and texts shall be individually illuminated.

Enclosures: Liquid oxygen tanks and other enclosures shall be illuminated in support of CCTV and visual surveillance without spillage into other areas onsite or offsite.

Trash: Collection areas shall be illuminated in service yards as a part of the yard illumination. Individual trash bins may not require illumination.

Loading docks and associated yards: Loading areas shall be fully illuminated for operations and in support of CCTV and other surveillance and Identification needs.

Building Entrances and Exits

Public Entrances And Lobbies

Public access to the facility should be restricted to a single or limited number of entrances.

Entrances

Public entrances: All public entrances to the In-Patient, Out-Patient, and Long-Term Care Facility shall have a screening vestibule that may be used when security requires individuals entering the building to pass through access control and screening prior to entering the building lobby. Perimeter doors should be locked after evening visiting hours are over, with entrance controlled by a security officer. Hospital staff should be allowed access by using swipe cards or similar controls.

Staff entrances: Staff entrances shall be located independently of main entrance lobbies and be convenient to staff parking.

Screening Vestibules

The screening vestibule shall have sufficient space and be provided with power, telecommunications and data connections for installation of access control and screening equipment that may be used should the need arise. Prevent access from drop-off to lobby in a straight line of travel, and provide sufficient size to accommodate several people with mobility aids.

For high-security facilities, vehicles may not approach within 50 feet (15 meters) of the entrance.

Doors: Entrance doors to the lobby shall be visible to or monitored by the security personnel in the main lobby and the Security Control Center.

Access within the facility: Access from the lobby to elevators, stairways and corridors shall be controlled through the use of electronic access control or mechanical locking devices, limiting access to specific floors and areas that house functions requiring restricted access.

- Install elevator call buttons requiring use of key cards or other electronic access control when they are located in restricted areas.

Access for Emergency Responders

The secure house key box for emergency responders or the Fire Command Center (FCC) shall be located near an entrance door at a location approved by the project manager. The door associated with the FCC shall be controlled and monitored by CCTV.

Structural: The entrance itself shall be constructed to fail in a way that subjects persons inside, or nearby, to as little hazard as possible.

- Protection of entrances and lobbies from vehicle ramming must be accomplished outside and in front of the entrance.
- If a covered drop-off area is provided, its supporting structure shall be independent of the main building and protected from intentional and unintentional damage by vehicles.
- Separate the public lobby from the adjacent hospital areas with partitions that extend to the underside of the floor above.

Façade: Glazing in the lobby area shall be laminated glass.

Doors and hardware: Exterior doors shall be in size, operation and other characteristics in compliance with applicable regulatory requirements. If doors are lockable, they shall comply with emergency egress requirements.

- Glass for entrance doors shall be laminated.
- Entrance doors shall be capable of being remotely locked and unlocked from the reception desk in the main lobby.

- Public entrance doors may be manually or power operated and may be swinging doors, horizontal sliding doors (power operated only) or revolving doors.

- Staff entrance doors shall prevent unauthorized access.

- Long-Term Care Unit shall be provided with electronic or mechanical locks on exterior doors, as well as visual monitoring and voice communication with connection to information desk or security office.

- Staff entrance door hardware shall include either mechanical or electronic locks.

- Means of egress doors that do not also function as entrances shall be provided with delayed action and alarmed emergency egress hardware.

Receptacles: Letter boxes and receptacles for trash and smoking paraphernalia shall not be located within five (5) feet (1.5 m) of load-bearing elements (load-bearing walls and columns, etc.). Those within 50 feet (15 m) of the building shall be designed to prevent depositing of explosive charges or to contain explosions with a charge weight.

Security Monitoring

At public entrances, create a "hard line" in the screening vestibule between the entrance and the lobby by providing a guard station with capacity to screen patients, visitors and packages when screening is required.

 Must Do ——————

All public entrances require security monitoring.

Security guard stations: Guard stations shall be located at building entrances available to the public. Guard stations shall be located where pedestrian traffic can be monitored and controlled by security personnel. If guard stations are located outside, they shall be protected from weather and capable of being secured when not in use.

- Security Control Center (SCC) shall be separated from public areas with Underwriter Laboratories (UL) Level 3 bullet-resistant construction which affords protection from most handguns.

- Guard stations that are not incorporated into an SCC shall be provided with a desk and capacity to communicate directly with the SCC.

- An intercom shall be provided from the front door to the guard station reception desk and SCC.

Screening devices: At all public entrances, where it may be necessary to screen all people entering a building, provide a screening vestibule. Provide the required connections for temporary installation of metal detectors and package screening equipment and sufficient space for their installation.

- Locate screening equipment in a manner that will prevent passage into the building or facility without passing through the devices.

- When screening devices are not permanently installed, provide secure storage in close proximity to their installation location.

- ▸ Locate screening equipment so as not to restrict emergency egress.
- ▸ **Security devices:** CCTV cameras shall be provided to monitor activities in the vestibules and lobbies of new and existing mission critical facilities and shall be located to provide views of approaching pedestrian and vehicular traffic, drop-off areas, building entrances, and departing pedestrian and vehicular traffic.

Patient Drop-Offs

Patient drop-offs shall be located at primary building entrances or other locations that will provide convenient access to services without hindering the flow of traffic. Patient drop-off areas shall not be located near staff-only entrances.

Vehicular Access

Drop-offs and staging areas for vehicles, including public transportation vehicles, shall be separated from the main building structure by at least 50 feet (15 meters).

Parking

Parking shall not be permitted in patient drop-off areas.

Building Exits And Life Safety Considerations

Means of egress shall not be obstructed by installation of security devices such as guard stations, screening equipment or other security devices. Delayed egress and alarmed exits shall comply with applicable codes and regulations.

Site Requirements

Provide an unobstructed and adequately lighted path from each means of egress to a safe location outside the building.

- ▸ Where the means of egress is accessible to persons with disabilities, provide an accessible route to a safe location outside the building.
- ▸ Where means of egress lead to loading docks or other service areas, direct users away from hazardous and pathological waste storage, mailrooms, and other areas that may be the source of injury or contamination.
- ▸ Plan and locate egress paths so that they are not obstructed by or with anti-ramming barriers or other similar devices.

Planning, Construction Details and Materials

Construction of building exits shall be consistent with the requirements for adjacent building envelope elements.

- ▸ Where laminated glass is required in nearby window openings, glazing for exit doors shall also be laminated.

- Where adjacent portions of the building require blast-resistant construction, construct the means of egress with a similar level of protection.

- Means of egress doors shall be of construction that makes unauthorized entry from the exterior difficult. Provide hardware that minimizes the opportunity for unauthorized entry by using components such as continuous hinges and astragals.

Security Monitoring

Where means of egress do not also function as access points for the building, provide card reader for authorized users and delayed-action, alarmed egress hardware to indicate unauthorized use.

- Provide CCTV cameras at locations with alarmed exits, at loading docks and other areas subject to pilferage.

- Install door status monitors at doors intended to be used only for emergency egress.

Functional Areas

Pharmacy caches located within the main facility shall be on a corridor leading to the loading dock, but no closer than 50 feet (15 m) to the loading dock or mailroom.

Entrances

Doors and frames to caches shall be opaque hollow metal, and shall be controlled and monitored.

Construction

Caches shall be enclosed in Class 1 fire-rated construction with surrounding construction 15-minute forced-entry resistant. Exterior construction shall be reinforced masonry or equivalent.

Partitions and openings: Interior partitions shall comply with the following when separating a cache from other building spaces, including corridors.

- Walls, floor and ceiling shall be permanently constructed and attached to each other. All construction, to include above a false ceiling and below a raised floor, shall be done in such a manner as to provide visual evidence of unauthorized penetration.

- Walls shall be reinforced, slab-to-slab, with nine-gauge expanded metal. The expanded metal shall be spot welded every six inches to vertical and horizontal metal supports of 16-gauge or greater thickness that has been solidly and permanently attached to the true floor and true ceiling.

- No windows or skylights shall be permitted in caches.

- Consider installing alarms.

HVAC: All vents, ducts and similar openings in excess of 96 square inches that enter or pass through a perimeter partition of the cache shall be protected with either bars or grills. If one dimension of the duct measures less than six inches or the duct is less than 96 square inches, bars are not required;

however, all ducts must be treated to provide sufficient sound attenuation. If bars are used, they must be a ½-inch in diameter, and steel welded vertically and horizontally six (6) inches on center; if grills are used, they must be of nine-gauge expanded steel.

- Openings in construction above ceilings or below raised-access floors shall be protected as previously described.

Electrical: All lighting, security devices and refrigerators within the cache shall be on emergency power.

Security

Entrance doors to the cache and vault doors, if any, within the cache shall be monitored by CCTV.

Computer Room

This section applies to the main computer room. In addition to the requirements of this section, NFPA 75: Protection of Electronic Computer/Data Processing Equipment shall apply.

Adjacencies

The main computer room shall be located not closer than 50 feet in any direction to main entrance lobbies, loading docks and mailrooms, and in no case directly above or below such spaces.

Entrances

Entrance doors to the main computer room and other computer rooms shall be controlled and monitored.

Construction

Surrounding walls and partitions shall be one-hour fire resistive construction and extend from slab to slab.

HVAC: All vents, ducts and similar openings in excess of 96 square inches that enter or pass through the perimeter of a computer room must be protected with either bars or grills. If one dimension of the duct measures less than six inches or duct is less than 96 square inches bars are not required; however, all ducts must be treated to provide sufficient sound attenuation.

If bars are used, they must be a ½-inch in diameter, and steel welded vertically and horizontally six inches on center; if grills are used, they must be of nine-gauge expanded steel.

- Openings in construction above ceilings or below raised-access floors shall be protected as previously described.

Security

All doors shall have motion-activated CCTV camera coverage on the egress side of the door.

Emergency Department

Vehicular Access: Only ambulances and emergency vehicles shall be allowed within 50 feet of the emergency department entrance. No other vehicles or traffic shall be allowed within 50 feet of the emergency department entrance. Are there special requirements in your state requiring you to post towing warning signs to allow you to tow cars that may have been abandoned during the emergency?

Drop-offs and staging areas for vehicles, including public transportation vehicles, shall be separated from the main building structure by at least 50 feet.

Entrances

Provide separate entrances for ambulatory patients and patients arriving by ambulance. In the event of a pandemic, you should consider separate entrances for well patients (i.e. broken arm or chest pain) versus those who may be affected by the virus.

Provide space for screening of pedestrians.

- ▸ Exterior doors: Entrances from the exterior shall be controlled and monitored.
- ▸ Interior entry doors: Entrances from the emergency (urgent care) area to the main building shall be solid core wood or hollow metal, and controlled and monitored.

Existing Facility – Entrances: Replace existing glass with laminated glass or install anti-fragmentation film on existing glass near the emergency department entrance.

Anti-ram barriers: Install stationary (passive) anti-ram barriers to prevent damage by vehicles approaching the emergency department entrance.

Façade: Provide laminated glass in doors and windows within 50 feet of the emergency department entrance.

Separate the treatment area and nurses' station from the waiting area and entrances with full-height construction.

HVAC: Locate all outdoor air intakes at least 100 feet from ambulance parking areas.

Security

You should have the capacity to screen patients, visitors and packages at the ambulatory patient entrance.

Exterior: Provide CCTV cameras capable of monitoring activity at the ambulance entrance and ambulance parking area and that display in the primary and secondary SCC.

CCTV: Provide CCTV monitoring of ER reception/waiting room and entrance from the exterior.

Intrusion detection: Provide door and lock status sensors and motion detectors in public toilets.

Duress alarm: Provide duress alarm for receptionist and at nurses' stations.

Emergency And/Or Stand-By Generator Room

Emergency and/or stand-by generators and related switchgear may be located in a separate structure from the main building or within the main building.

Elevation: Louvers protect from horizontal and vertical rain. The generator room shall not be located at an elevation subject to flooding at any time. Refer to the FEMA flood map for information.

Location in building: If within a main building such as a medical center, the generator room shall not be located closer than 50 feet of a loading dock/receiving area or mailroom, and shall not be located beneath such facilities.

HVAC: Areaways and louver openings serving the generator shall not open to the service yard for the loading dock. This includes all air intakes per NIOSH's recommendations to prevent individuals placing items in the HVAC unit and contaminating buildings or parts of the building.

Entrances

Exterior doors: Entrances from the exterior shall not open to the loading dock service yard. Doors shall be hollow metal, and controlled and monitored.

Interior entry doors: Entrances from the interior of the building shall be two-hour fire resistive construction and shall be controlled and monitored.

Construction

Emergency and/or stand-by generators and related switchgear shall be surrounded by one-hour fire resistive construction.

Security

Generators shall be monitored in the security control room, as well as at the engineering control center.

Energy Center/Boiler Plant

The energy center/boiler plant may be located within a main building or in an independent building.

Elevation: The energy center/boiler plant, including emergency and/or stand-by generators and switchgear, and engineering control center and access to fuel tanks, shall not be located at an elevation subject to flooding at any time. Refer to the FEMA flood map for information.

Location in building: If within a main building, such as a medical center, the energy center/boiler plant shall not be located closer than 50 feet of a loading dock/receiving area or mailroom and shall not be located beneath such facilities.

HVAC: Areaways and louver openings serving the energy center/boiler plant shall not open to the service yard for the loading dock and mailroom.

Entrances

The energy center/boiler plant shall not be entered from the service yard for the loading dock and/ or mailroom. Wherever possible the mailroom should have its own dedicated exhaust in case of contaminated packages, i.e., containing anthrax spores.

▸ Doors from the exterior to the energy center shall be controlled and monitored.

▸ Doors from the energy center to the interior of a main building shall be controlled and monitored.

Security

CCTV shall be provided to monitor any entrance to the energy center/boiler plant from the exterior.

Loading Dock and Service Entrances

Loading docks shall be adjacent to, but structurally separate from any facility. Loading docks may be located immediately adjacent to the following areas:

▸ Service yard

▸ Trash containers

▸ Freight elevators

▸ Non-critical bulk storage

▸ Mailroom

▸ Non-critical support areas such as laundries and maintenance spaces.

Loading docks shall not be located adjacent to or within 50 feet of the following.

▸ Fire Control Centers

▸ Security Control Center and Police Command Center

▸ Emergency or stand-by generators

▸ UPS

▸ Water storage – domestic and fire

▸ Main electrical switchgear

▸ Main utility service entrances

▸ Emergency egress from main building

▸ Childcare/development centers

▸ Flammable liquids or gas storage

▸ Outdoor air intakes

▸ **Coordination with vivarium:** Research animals and animal pathological waste shall have separate loading dock facilities, but may be served by the same service yard as the general loading dock.

Entrances

Pedestrian doors, stairs and ramps associated with loading docks shall be restricted to authorized personnel and be separated from the loading platform by not less than four (4) feet to discourage by-passing the entry door controls through the loading platform and other doors.

Provide electronic locks and door status monitors on doors serving loading docks.

▸ Exterior doors: Exterior pedestrian entrance doors and frames shall be constructed of heavy-duty hollow metal and shall be controlled and monitored.

▸ Interior entry doors: Doors and frames from the mailroom to the interior of the building shall be two-hour fire resistive construction and controlled and monitored.

Construction

Structural: Structure shall be designed to sustain an explosion from a charge weight (defined in the Physical Security Design Standards Data Definitions) within the loading dock and receiving area, as directed by the project manager.

Interior partitions: The loading dock and receiving area shall be separated from the corridors and spaces adjoining with reinforced masonry walls and doors of hollow metal construction and controlled and monitored.

Secured storage: Provide secure storage areas for delivered items awaiting uncrating and distribution within the facility and for hazardous and pathological waste.

HVAC: Locate all outdoor air intakes at least 100 feet (31 m) horizontally and 30 feet vertically from parking areas or on roof away from the roof line. Air serving the loading dock and receiving areas shall not circulate to other parts of the building.

Security

A minimum of 400 sq. ft. shall be provided within the receiving area for inspection and imaging of goods received.

Exterior: Install CCTV cameras to provide surveillance of all loading dock areas, including the gate, vehicle inspection areas, service yard and various containers, parked vehicles, loading and unloading activities and building entrances at the loading dock.

CCTV: The loading dock, including vehicles parked at the dock, shall be monitored by CCTV.

Access control: Dock lift controls shall be secured with a card-reader device to prevent unauthorized use for entry.

Loading docks shall be served from service yards enclosed by a secure fence or wall and power-operated sliding gate, controlled by card-access device and/or remote release and operation by a guard, the dock manager or other authorized person with intercom and CCTV ID.

Vehicle access: Vehicle access to the loading dock shall be restricted.

▸ Approaches to loading docks shall be configured to minimize the possibility of high-speed approach by any type of vehicle.

▸ Where the entrance gate to a service yard is directly from a public right-of-way, deployable vehicle barriers shall be provided on the inside of the gate, and shall be integrated with gate controls.

▸ Provide an area for the inspection of delivery vehicles that will not interfere with the flow of traffic on public rights of way, the site or the loading area.

Service yards: The yard shall be segregated from other vehicle and pedestrian traffic areas by screen walls.

▸ Delivery vehicle maneuvering and parking shall be within an enclosed service yard accessed by delivery vehicle roadways leading directly from the site perimeter.

▸ Trash, medical/pathological waste, and other containers, compactors and other similar equipment shall be located within the enclosed service yard and under CCTV surveillance.

Mailroom

Mailrooms may be located in the main building or in a separate structure on the site shared with loading dock, storage and other non-critical functions. When planning new mailrooms, they should their own dedicated HVAC. Mailrooms within the main building shall be located on an exterior wall.

Location: Mailrooms within the main building shall be located on an exterior wall and adjacent to the loading dock. Mailrooms may be located immediately adjacent to the following areas:

▸ Service yard

▸ Trash containers

▸ Loading dock

▸ Freight elevators

▸ Non-critical bulk storage

▸ Non-critical support areas such as laundries and maintenance spaces

Mailrooms shall not be located adjacent to or within 50 feet of the following:

▸ Fire Control Centers

▸ Security Control Center and Police Command Center

▸ Emergency or stand-by generators

▸ UPS

▸ Water storage – domestic and fire

▸ Main electrical switchgear

▸ Main utility service entrances

▸ Emergency egress from the main building

- ‣ Childcare/development centers
- ‣ Flammable liquids or gas storage
- ‣ Outdoor air intakes
- ‣ Dedicated exhausts

Entrances

Exterior doors: Exterior entrance doors and frames shall be constructed of heavy-duty hollow metal, and shall be controlled and monitored.

Interior entry doors: Doors and frames from the mailroom to the interior of the building shall be two-hour fire resistive construction, and controlled and monitored.

When located within the main building, structural columns passing through the mailroom and inspection area and floor slabs above them shall be structurally hardened to sustain an explosion within the mailroom or inspection area from a charge weight (defined in the Physical Security Design Standards Data Definitions) as directed by the project manager.

Mailboxes: Mailboxes, when provided, shall be in a separate room from the mailroom and inspection area, and shall comply with the mounting heights and other regulations of the U.S. Postal Service.

Interior partitions: The mailroom shall be separated from the mailbox room, corridors and spaces adjoining with reinforced masonry walls and doors of hollow metal construction.

Security

A minimum of 400 sq. ft. shall be provided within the receiving area for inspection and imaging of mail received. This may be space shared with the loading dock inspection area.

CCTV: The mailroom, including the inspection area and the exterior loading area serving the mailroom shall be monitored by CCTV.

Additional Requirements

Air serving the mailroom shall not circulate to other parts of the building.

Pharmacy

Deliveries to and shipments from pharmacies may be via the main loading dock and service yard. Pharmacies shall not be immediately adjacent to the loading dock or mailroom. Provide CCTV monitoring of pharmacy dispensing area, vault entrance and controlled-substance storage.

Other Areas

- ‣ Security staff should accompany the delivery of radioisotopes to nuclear medicine or radiology oncology treatment areas.
- ‣ Monitoring is needed for oxygen tank and bulk liquid oxygen storage areas.
- ‣ Fuel storage areas.

- Biohazardous waste storage.

- Awareness that hospitals have a number of potentially hazardous materials in various departments, including pharmaceuticals, antineoplastic drugs, anesthetic gases, lab specimen solvents, formaldehyde, xylene and others.

Source: Occupational Safety & Health Administration Technical Manual. Hospital Health Hazards. U.S. Department of Labor, www.osha.gov/dts/osta/otm/otm_vi/otm_vi_1.html.

Security Control Center (SCC)

The SCC shall provide continuous and consistent monitoring, surveillance, response and operation of security subsystems. The SCC shall be located in an area that is within the first level of security defense defined by the emergency preparedness plan. The SCC shall also be located above any potential flood areas such as the basement. The SCC shall be located:

- In an area that is within the first level of security defense defined by the emergency preparedness plan

- Above any potential flood areas, such as the basement

- In an area free of background noise influences that could impact equipment and SCC operations

- In an area capable of sending and receiving communication transmissions

- Away from exterior building walls that are adjacent to roadway traffic, parking, air intake areas or facility utility, environmental and operational areas, which if compromised, damaged or destroyed, could impact SCC operations, staff safety and their health

A secondary or backup SCC shall be established in another building (the same with the hospital's Call Center and Command Center) or location within the same facility that is far removed from the primary SCC. The secondary SCC shall be provided with full redundancy of the electronic security systems and associated security console operations.

The security technology shall be designed and engineered to provide flexibility to monitor and operate security subsystems from remote and multiple facility locations and security workstations. The SCC should follow ADA accessibility standards for approach, entry and exit access.

The SCC shall have physical security safeguards. The main entry door shall have a card reader or biometric security credential device for authorized personnel and an intercom or similar device for unauthorized persons to request assistance. Provide a fixed CCTV camera connected to a dedicated monitor within the SCC for direct communications and visual verification of the person using the intercom. Remote unlocking of the door shall be prohibited.

The size of the SCC shall be defined by the number of console bays required to house and operate the security subsystems and provide adjacency to where the security/police operations are. The SCC and security console power shall be provided from a dedicated security system power panel. The panel shall be connected to a backup power source capable of providing continuous power seven days a week for 24 hours a day. All field-mounted security equipment and security closets that interconnect and are monitored by the SCC and surge-protection at the equipment head-end shall be provided with backup power. There shall be a main power cut-off switch for the SCC equipment located inside the SCC.

Lighting shall be adequate and not cast shadows or create a glare that will reduce the security console operator's ability to monitor security console equipment. All fixtures shall also be on backup generator power. Finally, special care and consideration shall be given to the use of incandescent and fluorescent lighting, wall-mounted battery-powered emergency lighting, and illumination to the console writing space.

The air quality and temperature within the SCC shall allow for a comfortable work environment for both personnel and the security equipment. Ventilation controls shall also be provided on a separate air handling system that provides an isolated supply and return system. The SCC shall have a dedicated thermostat control unit and cut-off switch to be able to shut off ventilation to the SCC in the event of a chemical, biological or radiological (CBR) event or other related emergency. It shall be located on the first floor of the main patient care building adjacent to the highest potential trouble area, such as admissions, emergency or urgent care room or lobby and shall be located to allow appropriate response and deployment to respond to a security-related event.

Holding room: Shall be located within or adjacent to the security operations room.

▸   An additional holding room may be located within or adjacent to a perimeter screening facility.

A backup location should also be available to dispatch from and make/receive calls in the event of the main location becoming uninhabitable.

Entrances

Operations room: Doors shall be from a corridor used only by staff, and shall be controlled and operated.

Holding room: Doors and frames shall be heavy-gauge hollow metal steel construction, and door hardware shall be 15-minute forced-entry rated controlled and monitored.

When the operations room is adjacent to or opens onto areas occupied by unscreened public, such as lobbies, emergency rooms and public corridors, construction, including partitions from slab to slab, doors, windows and other openings separating the unit from such spaces, shall be one-hour fire resistive, UL level 3 ballistic-resistant.

CCTV surveillance shall be provided of the entire room through an opening glazed with transparent polycarbonate in a steel frame firmly anchored to the wall. If requested by the project manager, the CCTV camera shall be covert and use lenses made for the purpose.

Records Storage and Archives

Records storage rooms shall be located not nearer than 50 feet in any direction from main entrance lobbies, loading docks and mailrooms, and in no case directly above or below such spaces. Ensure offsite storage of back up computer tapes.

Entrances

Entrances to archival storage spaces, including book stacks, computer main frames, and valuable or historical records and collections shall be controlled and monitored.

▸ Emergency egress doors from archival storage spaces shall be controlled and monitored, and shall have motion-activated CCTV camera coverage of the egress side of the door with all device monitors at a central location within the archival or library area.

Construction

Records storage rooms shall comply with National Archives and Records Administration (NARA) Facility Standards for Records Storage Facilities – Part 1228, Subpart K.

▸ Where electronic media or data storage facilities are essentially computer rooms, the area shall comply with the requirements of section 5.4.

Security

Archives for rare and valuable artifacts and documents shall be provided with motion detectors and CCTV. A good recommendation is to have about 30 days of storage capability on voice recording and CCTV systems, and for visitor badge programs, one year of storage of images and data.

Building Envelope

Walls

Non-load Bearing Walls

Walls shall be designed to suffer damage but sustain only modest deformation in response to the calculated peak pressures and impulses resulting from the design-level vehicle threat located at the stand-off distance.

Supporting structure: Walls shall span from slab to slab and shall not be attached directly to gravity load-bearing elements (such as columns and shear walls) unless an advanced analysis of the load-bearing element demonstrates it can accept the maximum forces of the members framing into it without compromising its capacity.

Loads: Walls shall be able to accept the tributary loads transferred from glazed fenestration, in addition to the design level pressures applied directly to their surface.

Façade Windows

All façade windows shall be designed to crack but fragments shall enter the occupied space and land on the floor no further than 10 feet (3 m) from the façade in response to the calculated peak pressures and impulses resulting from the design-level vehicle threat located at the stand-off distance.

Glass: Windows shall be constructed using debris mitigating materials such as laminated glass.

Glazing: The glass shall be restrained within the mullions with a sufficient bite or structural silicone adhesive to allow it to develop its post-damage capacity.

Mullions: Mullions are vertical structures which divide and may strengthen adjacent window units or provide structural support within doors. They shall be designed to accept the design-level pressures while sustaining only slight deformations.

Curtain wall: A Curtain wall is an outer covering of a building in which the outer walls are non-structural, but serve to keep out the weather, specifically to resist air or water infiltration and sway from wind or seismic forces. Framing members shall span from slab to slab and shall not be attached directly to gravity load-bearing elements (such as columns and shear walls) unless an advanced analysis of the load-bearing element demonstrates it can accept the maximum forces of the members framing into it without compromising its load-bearing capacity.

Atria

All vertical glass surfaces shall be designed to crack, but fragments shall enter the occupied space and land on the floor no further than 10 feet (3 m) from the façade in response to the calculated peak pressures and impulses resulting from the design-level vehicle threat located at the stand-off distance.

Skylights: Skylights shall be designed to crack, but remain in its frame in response to the calculated peak pressures and impulses resulting from the design-level vehicle threat located at the stand-off distance.

Glass: Atria shall be constructed using debris mitigating materials such as laminated glass.

Glazing: The glass shall be restrained within the mullions with a sufficient bite or structural silicone adhesive to allow it to develop its post-damage capacity.

Mullions: The mullions shall be designed to accept the design-level pressures while sustaining only slight deformations.

Framing: Atria framing members shall be designed to continue carrying gravity loads while sustaining maximum allowable deformations.

Roof Structure

Roof structure shall be designed to withstand the design-level vehicle threat located at the stand-off distance, while sustaining only slight deformation. The blast loading shall take into account the presence of parapets (wall-like barriers at the edge of a roof, terrace, balcony or other structure), the diffusion of blast waves and the spatial extent of the roof surface.

Skylights

Skylights shall be designed to crack, but remain in its frame in response to the calculated peak pressures and impulses resulting from the design-level vehicle threat located at the stand-off distance.

Glazing: Skylight glass shall be restrained within the mullions with a sufficient bite or structural silicone adhesive to allow it to develop its post-damage capacity.

Mullions: The mullions shall be designed to accept the design-level pressures while sustaining slight deformations.

Penthouses Enclosing Mission Critical Equipment

Penthouse façade shall be designed to withstand the effects of hurricane wind loads and debris impact. Penthouse enclosures shall also be designed to resist the design-level vehicle threat located at the stand-off distance to be consistent with the hardened intakes and exhausts.

Air Intakes and Exhausts

Air intakes and exhausts shall be designed to minimize the blast over pressure admitted into critical spaces to the design-level vehicle threat located at the stand-off distance by means of hardened plenums and structured baffles. The design shall deny a direct line of sight from the design-level vehicle threat located at the stand-off distance to the critical infrastructure within.

Entrances and lobbies: Maintain positive pressure in lobbies and entrance areas.

Locate all outdoor air intakes a minimum of 100 feet from areas where vehicles may be stopped with their engines running. Locate all outdoor air intakes a minimum of 30 feet above finish grade or on roof away from the roof line and away from areas where something can be introduced into the air intake.

Hurricane areas: Louvers in areas prone to hurricanes or wind-debris hazards shall be certified by the manufacturer to meet the following: the Uniform Static Air Pressure Test, Cyclic Wind Pressure Test, Large Missile Impact Test and Wind Driven Rain Resistance Test.

Utilities

Utility Entrances

Mechanical

Alternate connections for steam and chilled water: Provide means for the connection of an alternate source, such as a mobile boiler or chiller.

Steam, chilled water, water, and fuel system distribution: Distribution systems shall be underground and shall be looped systems, such that an interruption at any one point can be isolated and service maintained to the facility. Piped utility systems, in particular fuel systems, shall include enhanced capability to resist external forces. Steam and condensate piping shall be installed above the flood zone.

Separation of sanitary sewer and storm drain systems: Sanitary sewer and storm drain systems shall be separate.

Manhole and handhole covers: Manholes and handholes shall be equipped with lockable covers.

Water service: Two independent sources are required. This may consist of two independent services from an offsite water provider or a single source from an offsite provider and an onsite water well with treatment means. Consider a non-potable well to allow flushing of toilets and other systems. You can install piping to upper floors so that you don't have to move potable five- gallon containers upstairs or in elevators – assuming the elevators are working.

Protection of utility-owned service equipment: Above-ground utility-owned service equipment shall be located within a building envelope when possible or be protected by limited-access masonry enclosures and be located a minimum of 100 feet in all directions from vulnerable areas. Coordinate with the serving utility.

Electrical

Number of services: Two separate electrical service feeders are required.

Separation of services: Electric service feeders shall be underground, located away from other utility services, and located away from vulnerable areas. Services shall be separated by a minimum distance of 100 feet.

Protection of utility-owned service equipment: Utility-owned service and metering equipment shall be located within a building envelope when possible or be protected by limited-access masonry enclosures and be located a minimum of 100 feet in all directions from vulnerable areas. Coordinate with the serving utility.

Separation of feeders: Feeders that form a primary selective pair shall not be located closer than 100 feet to each other, shall be encased in concrete, and shall enter served buildings at different locations. Feeder entry points will maintain a minimum distance of 100 feet or greater in all directions from areas such as loading docks or similar defined areas of vulnerability.

Location of distribution equipment: All electrical distribution components, such as medium- and low-voltage switchgear and transformers, shall be located within a building envelope.

Manhole and handhole covers: Manholes and handholes shall be equipped with lockable covers.

Telecommunications

Number of services: Two services from each telecommunications provider are required, preferably with delivery from different central offices or sites.

Separation of services: Telecommunications cable pathways shall be underground, located away from other utility services, and located away from vulnerable areas. Where more than one service is obtained, services shall be separated by a minimum distance of 100 feet.

Telecommunications systems distribution: An underground ring topology shall be used for telecommunications cable pathways that connect multiple buildings. This will provide two underground pathways for telecommunications services to all buildings. Sizing of conduits shall be based on a 40-percent fill, and there will be a minimum of two spare four-inch (100 mm) conduits between buildings. Conduits shall be encased in concrete. Distance between manholes or handholes shall not be greater than 400 feet.

Separation of pathways: Ring distribution pathways shall not be located closer than 100 feet to each other. Pathways shall enter served buildings at different locations and shall not be exposed on the building exterior. Quantity and size of conduits shall be determined by site design.

Telecommunications entry points shall maintain a minimum distance of 100 feet or greater in all directions from areas such as loading docks or similar defined areas of vulnerability.

Location of telecommunications equipment: All telecommunications components other than inter-building cabling shall be located within the building envelope.

Manhole and handhole covers: Manholes and handholes shall be equipped with lockable covers.

Energy Center

Requirements

The energy center contains utility production and distribution equipment, as well as incoming services from offsite utility providers, and is responsible for providing utility services during normal operating conditions, as well as during and after natural and manmade disaster events. The utility services feeding into the energy center include but may not be limited to electricity, potable water, natural gas and fuel oil. The utilities feeding to and/or from the energy center and the mission critical facility shall be electricity, steam and condensate return, and chilled water supply and return.

Sustained Service

The energy center shall sustain utility services for a minimum time period of four (4) days.

Stand-by Power

Paralleled diesel generators shall provide complete stand-by power to the energy center and may provide full stand-by power to other buildings.

Long-replacement-time Equipment

For equipment that has a long replacement time, provide for additional physical protection and/or installation of redundant equipment or connections that will alleviate extended shutdown time.

Water And Fuel Storage

Requirements

Storage shall be provided for potable and industrial water, fire protection, wastewater and contaminated water, and fuels for use during the period under which offsite utilities are unavailable. At a minimum, water and generator fuel storage shall support four (4) days of operation, and boiler fuel storage shall support 10 January days of operation.

Storage Volume Criteria

Water: Minimum criteria to be used in determining storage requirements are:

▸ **Potable water:** In Florida, the rule of thumb is one gallon per shift per day for staff, three gallons per shift per day per patient – so a risk assessment needs to be done.

▸ **Industrial water:** Industrial water requirements include cooling tower and boiler make-up water. A peak summer and winter consumption shall be normalized over a seven-day period. The profile with the greatest consumption shall be used to determine industrial water storage requirements.

▸ **Wastewater retention:** 40 gal/day/person.

▸ **Fire protection water:** Minimum of 120,000 gallons, and when unfavorable conditions occur, minimum fire demand shall not be less than 180,000 gallons. NFPA 1 requirements apply in all cases.

▸ **Contaminated water:** Minimum 5,000 gallons of holding capacity for water contaminated with hazardous material(s).

▸ Capacity to treat non-potable or use non-potable water.

Generator Fuel: A peak summer and winter consumption profile shall be normalized over a seven-day period. The profile with the greatest consumption shall be used to determine generator fuel storage requirements.

Boiler Fuel: Onsite boiler fuel storage in the amount necessary for 10 January days of operation is required.

Water Storage Emergency Connection

The water storage system shall include emergency connections to allow for a change in supply source or change in delivery points.

Water Treatment

Provide water treatment equipment to mitigate from environmental contaminants including, but not limited to, fungi, dust, debris, outside condensation and corrosion.

Onsite Water Well

Where available, use an onsite water well as an alternate source for potable, industrial and/or fire protection water.

Protection of Equipment

Protect all water and fuel storage, pumping, metering and regulating equipment with screen walls or barriers. All tanks shall remain functional and accessible during emergencies. Tanks shall be water tight and secured to prevent buoyancy. Intakes and vents shall be located above the base flood elevation, unobstructed and in areas not subject to flooding.

Building Systems

HVAC

Locate major mechanical equipment above the ground floor in an area not subject to flooding.

Emergency connections: Include emergency connections for chilled water and steam services at or near the building entrance point, where it will be unobstructed and accessible in an area not subject to flooding. Where looped systems enter the building at two points, the emergency connections need only be installed on one entry.

Security Control Center (SCC): In the SCC, provide a display-only terminal, which will display status and alarm conditions reported by the energy center, the building(s) environmental control system(s), medical gas and vacuum system alarms, stand-by and/or emergency generators and other similar systems.

Entrances and lobbies: Maintain positive pressure in lobbies and entrance areas.

Intakes and Exhausts

Outdoor air intakes: All air intakes shall be located so that they are protected from external sources of contamination. Locate the intakes away from publicly accessible areas, minimize obstructions near the intakes that might conceal a device, and use intrusion alarm sensors to monitor the intake areas.

▸ Locate all outdoor air intakes a minimum of 100 feet from areas where vehicles may be stopped with their engines running.

▸ Locate all outdoor air intakes a minimum of 30 feet above finish grade or on roof away from the roof line.

Air intakes and exhausts: Design to minimize the blast over pressure admitted into critical spaces and to deny a direct line of sight from a vehicle threat located at the stand-off distance to the critical infrastructure within.

Hurricane areas: Louvers in areas prone to hurricanes or wind-debris hazards shall be certified by the manufacturer to meet the following Florida Building Code tests: Uniform Static Air Pressure Test, Cyclic Wind Pressure Test, Large Missile Impact Test and Wind Driven Rain Resistance Test.

Electrical Systems

Stand-by Power Systems

Generators are required to provide power for the entire mission critical facility load. The stand-by power system is not identical to the NFPA-required emergency power system, which supplies power to a specifically mandated set of health care facility loads. The stand-by power system is in addition to the emergency power system.

Stand-by generators: Generators shall be diesel compression engine type. Generators should provide power at the highest practical voltage level, preferably the medium-voltage utility service entrance voltage, and be paralleled into the normal power electrical system at a point as close as possible to the utility service entrance. An assumed peak load of 10 watts per gross square foot of building area is suggested for sizing the capacity of the generator(s). Generators, paralleling equipment, and associated fuel and electrical components shall be located in dedicated structures or rooms. Stand-by power systems shall be located a minimum distance of 100 feet or greater in all directions from areas such as loading docks or similar defined areas of vulnerability.

Load shedding controls: Automatic controls shall selectively shed load from the stand-by power system upon failure of one or more stand-by generators to operate. The last loads to be shed shall be the "normal" sources for the emergency electrical system automatic transfer switches.

Emergency connections: Include emergency connections for emergency and stand-by generators at or near the building entrance point. Where looped systems enter the building at two points, the emergency connections need only be installed on one entry.

Uninterruptible Power Systems (UPS)

Provide UPS equipment for mission critical telecommunications equipment. The telecommunications facilities include the entrance facility (DEMARC), main telephone room and main computer room. UPS equipment and its associated power distribution unit (PDU) are essential pieces of bridging equipment, used during the time gap between loss of utility power and energization of the emergency or stand-by generator systems. They are also intended to provide time for an orderly shutdown of equipment in the event stand-by generators do not operate properly.

Modularity: Where multiple UPS are used, they shall be identically sized to allow for interchangeability.

Space for UPS: Provide required UPS floor space in rooms which require UPS-backed power.

Battery runtime: Size battery systems for a minimum of 20 minutes of full rated output. Individual project needs may dictate a longer runtime.

Telephone Equipment Room

The telephone equipment room shall house the main telephone switching equipment for the facility and contain public address system equipment, interconnection to the portable radio system and other equipment that interconnects with the telephone system. The telephone equipment room must be located in a secure area of the building on the ground floor or higher. The room shall not be located within 25 feet of an outside wall or delivery area and shall not be located directly below laboratories, kitchens, laundries, toilets, showers or other areas where water service is provided.

HVAC: The telephone equipment room must be provided with generator-backed HVAC service.

Power: All equipment in the telephone equipment room must be powered from either a building or local UPS that will provide a minimum of four (4) hours of service at full rated output.

Conduit pathways: Conduit pathways used to interconnect the main telephone room, the demarcation point or DEMARC room and the main computer room must be configured in a ring topology to provide two pathways to any of the three locations.

Main Computer Room

The main computer room contains all of the main data processing equipment for the mission critical facility. The main computer room shall not be located adjacent to the main telephone room and shall not be located directly below laboratories, kitchens, laundries, toilets, showers or other areas where water service is provided.

HVAC: The main computer room must be provided with generator-backed HVAC service.

Power: All equipment in the main computer room must be powered from either a building or local UPS that will provide a minimum of 20 minutes of service at full-rated output.

Telecommunications Distribution Rooms

Telecommunications distribution rooms are located on all floors of the building and distribute telephone, data and other telecommunications to work spaces located throughout the building.

Telecommunications distribution rooms shall be centrally located on the floors so that cables connecting workstations are no longer than 295 feet. In many cases, this will require more than one distribution room on the floor. Telecommunications distribution rooms must be stacked vertically.

HVAC: Telecommunications distribution rooms must be provided with generator-backed HVAC service.

Power: All equipment in the telecommunications distribution rooms must be powered from either a building or local UPS that will provide a minimum of 20 minutes of service at full rated output.

WLAN System

A wireless data system facilitates rapid restoration of limited data communications services in the building after a catastrophic event. Provide a wireless data access system, or install infrastructure (cabling) placed for later system installation. Provisions shall be made during the initial telecommunications system design and installation to implement a wireless data system throughout the building. These provisions are required whether a wireless data system will be initially installed or not. Specific design requirements will include placement of data access points, plans to interface with antenna distribution system, and equipment space and power requirements in telecommunications distribution rooms.

System design must include provision for PoE (Power over Ethernet) to supply power to any individual access points. Horizontal cabling used to connect Wireless Access Points (WAPs) shall be the same type as cable used for other building wireless access points. Wireless LAN access points distributed throughout the facility must be secured to the ceiling or building in a way that requires a special tool for removal. Data security on the WLAN must be implemented using the most secure industry standard at the time the system is actually put in operation. System design must include the ability for the wireless data system to use the building distributed antenna system, if available, for distributing data signals.

Portable Radio System

Provide a portable radio system. The portable radio system provides radio paging for security services and facilities management services both inside buildings and throughout the campus, where there are multiple buildings. All fixed radio equipment must be mounted according to manufacturer's recommendations, and mounting provisions must comply with applicable seismic requirements.

Radio equipment may be located in a penthouse or one of the telecommunication distribution rooms. The location must be coordinated with access to both the antenna equipment and the vertical riser (telecommunications distribution room) spaces. A penthouse may allow weather to impact the devices, so an internal space may be preferable. Don't forget alternative systems including space for HAM radios, hard wired and portable satellite phones, and 800 MHZ radios to communicate with local law enforcement, fire or other local emergency management.

HVAC: Fixed radio equipment must be provided with generator-backed HVAC service.

Power: Fixed radio equipment must be powered from either a building or local UPS that will provide a minimum of 24 hours of service at full rated output. Some hospital command centers have even hard-wired a connection to their generator room.

Satellite Radiotelephone System

Provide a satellite radiotelephone system. The purpose of the satellite radiotelephone is to provide a very basic and limited telephone capability in the event internal and external phone systems failure. The satellite radiotelephone must be able to make local, long distance and international telephone calls directly over a satellite connection without using any land facilities.

Public Address System

The public address (PA) system is defined as an emergency communication life safety system by the National Fire Protection Association (NFPA). The all-call paging function for hospital emergency codes and interconnection to the facility's NFPA-identified critical care telephone system elevates classification of the system's emergency communication rating to critical care. Therefore, installation and operation shall adhere to all appropriate national, federal, and life safety and support codes, the more stringent of which shall govern.

All cabling and installation practices associated with equipment intended for use in a critical care facility will be adhered to. The PA system must be able to be overridden by security personnel during an extraordinary event. All central PA equipment shall be located in the main telephone room to facilitate interconnection with the telephone system.

Power: PA system equipment must be powered from either a building or local UPS that will provide a minimum of four (4) hours of service at full rated output.

Consider standardizing or adopting standardized emergency codes.

Distributed Antenna System

Provide a distributed antenna system in the facility. The distributed antenna system works in conjunction with the various radio systems in the building to improve portable radio system coverage in the building and provides the ability to use one common antenna system for multiple services. Services that may be supported include the portable radio system, public safety radio rebroadcast, cellular radio system rebroadcast and support for WLAN data service. All distributed antenna system equipment shall be located in the telecommunications distribution rooms.

Power: Distributed antenna system equipment must be powered from either a building or local UPS that will provide a minimum of four (4) hours of service at full-rated output.

Cabling: Comply with all optical fiber, coaxial, and antenna system cabling and installation practices associated with cabling intended for use in a critical care facility.

VSAT Satellite Data Terminal

A Very Small Aperture Terminal (VSAT) data terminal acts as a backup data system and provides limited data capability if all ground-based services were to fail. It provides a data capability that is not dependent on local service providers. VSAT equipment is roof-mounted and interfaces with data translation equipment located in the main computer room.

Power: VSAT equipment must be powered from either a building or local UPS that will provide a minimum of 20 minutes of service at full-rated output.

Plumbing Systems

Medical Air and Oxygen Systems

Medical air and oxygen systems shall be secured to prevent unauthorized tampering, contaminating, or cross-connecting of systems.

Fire Protection Systems

Fire Department Hose Connections

Fire department hose connections located on the exterior of a building shall be secured in a suitable enclosure that limits access to authorized personnel. Coordinate with the serving fire department.

Security Systems

CCTV Monitoring And Surveillance (CCTV)

This section addresses physical security standards for the two basic uses of a video surveillance, or CCTV, system: access control and general surveillance. It describes the selection, application and performance of the CCTV system, which includes cameras, monitors, controlling and recording equipment, and centralized management and operations of the system.

The CCTV system shall be used to monitor building entrances, restricted areas, mission critical asset areas and alarm conditions. The CCTV system shall be used for surveillance and observations of defined exterior areas, such as site and roadway access points, parking lots, perimeter of the building and interior areas, from a centralized Security Control Center (SCC).

System compatibility: All components of the CCTV system shall be fully compatible and shall not require the addition of interface equipment or software upgrades to ensure a fully operational system. The CCTV system shall be able to be fully integrated with other security subsystems.

Networked versus Stand-alone CCTV System

The CCTV system shall be designed and engineered as either a networked or stand-alone system.

Networked CCTV system: A networked CCTV system shall be utilized when multiple cameras, monitors, controllers and recording devices are configured to make up what is defined as a whole CCTV system. All components of the system shall be monitored and controlled at a single point, the SCC, using either a matrix switcher or a desktop computer.

Stand-alone CCTV system: A stand-alone CCTV system may be used for a single application and designated location use only and may complement the physical access control system (PACS) for a specific area. Fixed camera(s) shall be positioned in a manner to allow viewing of specific entry control point(s) through the use of a dedicated CCTV system monitor located in a common viewing area.

Cameras

The design, installation and use of CCTV cameras shall support the visual identification and surveillance of persons, vehicles, assets, incidents and defined locations. All cameras shall meet the following requirements.

▸ Cameras shall be charge coupled device (CCD) cameras and conform to National Television System Committee (NTSC) formatting criteria.

▸ Cameras shall be color and programmable to digitally switch from color to black and white at dusk and vice versa at dawn.

▸ Cameras shall be rated for continuous operation.

▸ Each camera function and activity shall be addressed within the system by a unique twenty (20) character user defined name. The use of codes or mnemonics identifying the CCTV action shall not be accepted.

▸ Cameras shall have built-in video motion detection that automatically monitors and processes activity information from each camera based upon how the surveillance field-of-view is programmed.

▸ When the camera is used as part of a CCTV system computer network, video encoder shall be used to convert the signal from the NTSC criteria to Moving Picture Experts Group (MPEG) format.

▸ All cameras shall be home run to a monitoring and recording device via controlling video equipment, such as a matrix switcher or network server that is monitored from a designated SCC location. The use of wireless cameras may also be considered.

▸ Fixed versus pan/tilt/zoom (P/T/Z) cameras: CCTV cameras may be either fixed or pan/tilt/zoom (P/T/Z).

▸ Fixed cameras shall be the primary means of surveillance to monitor designated access control and monitoring points.

▸ P/T/Z cameras shall complement the use of fixed cameras when large and multiple areas of surveillance are required and using video motion detection provides additional surveillance advantages.

▸ P/T/Z cameras shall be used and deployed for all site perimeter and exterior building areas.

▸ Fixed cameras shall be used to monitor interior building areas; P/T/Z cameras may be used to provide supplemental surveillance coverage of building interiors, where necessary.

Hardwired versus wireless cameras: CCTV cameras, classified as hardwired, directly connect to a monitoring device using video signal imaging cable. A wireless CCTV camera application is directly connected via a remote receiver that requires constant line-of-sight communications with the camera and the monitoring device.

▸ Hardwired or IP cameras shall be the preferred method of installation.

▸ Hardwired cameras shall be connected to the monitoring equipment with continuous wiring used as the media transmission system.

▸ Prior to selection of wireless cameras consider the potential effects, such as geographical area of coverage, environmental interference and distance from the monitoring location, that impacts the use of this technology.

Color versus black and white cameras: All CCTV cameras shall be color that allows for black and white applications.

▸ Cameras shall be able to switch between color and black and white through a programmable feature built into the camera.

▸ Color shall be the primary mode automatically switching to black and white when light levels drop below normal specifications.

▸ Cameras will be set to black and white on a full-time basis only when installed in a low-light level that requires the camera to operate at a higher resolution than normal.

Camera lenses: CCTV camera lenses shall be used in a manner that provides maximum coverage of the area being monitored and shall meet the following requirements:

▸ Two types of lenses shall be used for both interior and exterior fixed cameras.

▸ Manual variable focus lenses shall be used in large areas monitored by the camera and shall allow for settings at any angle of field to maximize surveillance coverage.

▸ Auto iris fixed lenses shall be used in areas where a small specific point of reference is monitored.

▸ Specific lens size shall be determined using a field-of-view calculation provided by the manufacture.

▸ There can be problems with day/night cameras and with digital cameras, as they pixilate.

▸ Camera enclosures: All cameras and lenses shall be enclosed in tamper-resistant housing.

▸ Both interior and exterior cameras shall be housed within a tamper-proof camera enclosure.

▸ Exterior camera enclosures shall be environmental proof to protect against unique weather elements associated with the specific facility geographical area.

Camera installation, mounts, poles and bases: All camera equipment shall be installed to ensure that all components are fully compatible as a system. Adhere to guidance provided by the National Electrical Contractors Association Standard, NECA 303-2005, Installing Closed-Circuit Television (CCTV) Systems.

▸ Camera mounts shall be installed on approved mounting surfaces structured for weight, wind load and extreme weather conditions.

▸ Camera mounts shall be installed in a manner that will not inhibit camera operation or field of view.

- Where camera is mounted to a rooftop or within a parapet, ensure that the mount is designed and installed in a manner that the equipment can be swiveled inward for maintenance and upkeep purposes.

- All camera poles shall be constructed of metal with a concrete base and shall be installed and grounded in accordance with the National Electrical Code (NEC).

- Camera poles shall be weather resistant.

- Camera pole heights shall be no less than 15 feet (4.6 m) and no greater than 50 feet high.

- Cameras and their mounts may share the same pole with lighting when the following conditions are met:

  ▷ A hardened wire carrier system is installed inside the pole to separate the high-voltage power cables for the lighting from the power and signal cables for the camera and mount.

  ▷ The camera and mount are installed and positioned in a manner that the lighting will not deter from, cause blind spots or shadows, and interfere with the video picture and signal.

  ▷ All camera poles and mounts shall be installed in locations that will allow for optimum view of the area of coverage.

Power source: All CCTV cameras and mounts shall be powered remotely by a UL-listed power supply unit (PSU) as follows.

- The PSU shall have the ability to power at least four exterior cameras or eight interior cameras.

- A backup direct power feed from a security system power panel shall be provided to the camera and mount. A step down transformer shall also be installed at the camera location to ensure a proper operating voltage is provided to the camera and mount.

- The CCTV system shall be supported by a UPS and/or dedicated stand-by generator circuit to ensure continuous operation of cameras, including all surveillance monitoring and recording equipment.

Lightning and surge protection: With the exception of fiber-optic cables, all cables and conductors that act as control, communication or signal lines shall include surge protection.

Site coordination: Site and building exterior lighting shall be coordinated and installed in a manner that allows the CCTV system to provide positive identification of a person, vehicle, incident and location.

- Lighting shall not provide bright illumination behind the main field of camera view.

- Cameras shall be installed in a manner that no lighting will point directly at the camera lens causing blind spots and blackouts.

- Provide routine maintenance of lighting systems and replacement of lighting fixtures and luminaries that are necessary for operational integrity of the CCTV system.

- CCTV cameras shall be installed so that landscaping will not deter from the intended field of view.

▸ Cameras shall not be mounted in trees, bushes or any other natural landscape that will in the long term degrade the view or operation of the CCTV system.

▸ Cameras shall not be installed behind, next to, or on any natural or manmade object that will restrict the field of view, cause signal loss or prevent the camera from being fully operational.

▸ Perform routine landscape maintenance that is necessary for operational integrity of the CCTV system.

Additional CCTV System Components

Monitors: All CCTV monitors shall be color and able to display analog, digital and other images in either NTSC or MPEG format associated with the operation of the Security Management System (SMS).

Matrix switcher/network server (controlling equipment): Controlling equipment shall be used to call up, operate and program all cameras associated with CCTV system components. Controlling equipment shall have the ability to operate the cameras locally and remotely. A matrix switcher or a network server shall be used as the CCTV system controller. The controlling equipment shall allow the transmission of live video, data, and audio over an existing Ethernet network or a dedicated security system network, requiring an IP address or Internet Explorer 5.5 or higher. The controlling equipment shall be able to perform as an analog-to-Ethernet "bridge," allowing for the control of matrices, multiplexers and P/T/Z cameras.

Keyboards and joysticks: A keyboard shall provide direct operator interface with the controlling equipment to allow for call-up, operation of cameras and mounts, and programming of controlling equipment, as well as cameras and monitors. Where a matrix switcher is used, ensure the keyboard is outfitted with a joystick to provide direct interface with CCTV camera controls.

Controlling and Recording Equipment

All cameras on the CCTV system shall be recorded in real time using a Digital Video Recorder (DVR), Network Video Recorder (NVR) or a Time Lapse Video Recorder (VCR). The type of recording device shall be determined by the size and type of CCTV system designed and installed, as well as the extent to which the system is to be used. Most facilities now use digital recording mediums. Have 30 days storage capacity, so you have ample time to discern criminal activity and take action.

NVR: The NVR shall be used within the CCTV system for large or small CCTV system set-ups. The NVR shall be used when the CCTV system is configured as part of the SMS only. Input to the NVR shall be considered when designing and installing all cameras that will be connected to the NVR.

Time lapse VCR: The time lapse VCR shall be used for all CCTV systems of fewer than 16 cameras that are not part of an SMS or connected to a CCTV system network.

▸ A time-lapse VCR using analog tapes shall have the capability to record on a continuous 24-hour basis.

▸ These recordings shall be stored in a dry, cool, central location that is secured and shall be maintained in accordance with police directives.

▸ The time-lapse VCR shall be used as a backup to DVR and NVR equipment.

▸ The goal should be to retain records for approximately 30 days.

Video Motion Detection

CCTV cameras shall have built-in video motion detection capability that automatically monitors and processes information from each CCTV camera. Cameras shall be programmed to automatically change viewing of an area of interest without human intervention and shall automatically record the activity until reset by the CCTV system operator.

Timing: This feature shall detect motion within the camera's field of view and provide the SCC monitors immediate automatic visual, remote alarms and motion-artifacts as a result of detected motion.

Interface with IDS: The video motion detection shall be interfaced with the intrusion detection system (IDS) to provide redundancy in the security alarm reporting system.

Other system interface: Cameras shall be designed to interface and respond to exterior and interior alarms, security phones/call-boxes, duress alarms and intercoms upon activation.

Intrusion Detection System (IDS)

The Intrusion Detection System (IDS) includes motion detection, glass break and door contact sensors, among other devices. These devices provide alternative methods to detect actual or attempted intrusion into protected areas through the use of alarm components, monitoring and reporting systems. The IDS shall have the capability of being integrated with DSPI, PACS and CCTV systems. All IDS shall meet UL 639 Intrusion Detection Standard.

System Elements and Features

IDS shall be used to monitor the site perimeter, building envelope and entrances, and interior building areas where access is restricted or controlled.

System Integration

IDS shall be able to be fully integrated with other security subsystems using direct hardwire or computer interface.

Planning and Selection Criteria

IDS shall provide multiple levels or points of detection as far away as possible from an asset to be protected. The type of IDS sensor to be used shall be determined by the criticalness of the asset to protect, size of the protected space, local threat assessment results and capability of the sensor.

Layout and zoning: Areas to be covered by sensors shall be charted and set up in protection or coverage zones prior to selection and placement of sensors. IDS devices of different technologies, such as motion detection, glass break and magnetic contacts, shall be zoned separately.

Physical environment: A survey shall be conducted to determine whether conditions exist that may adversely affect the sensors and cause them not to detect within their performance limits or to cause false alarms.

▸ For exterior applications consider the effects of foliage, rain, fence fabric, underground utilities and other environmental conditions.

▸ Interior applications of sensors shall consider HVAC location, heat sources, transient light, vibration, moving machinery, dust and humidity.

Networked versus Stand-alone

Networked: IDS devices shall be networked when multiple sensors and controllers are being utilized. All components of the IDS shall be monitored and controlled at a single point.

Stand-alone: Stand-alone IDS shall be used for single office space only as determined by the project manager and shall be a means to complement the physical access control system (PACS) and CCTV system.

Hardwired versus Wireless

Hardwired alarms: All sensors and controllers shall be hardwired and directly connected to the local controller, keypad or other security subsystems using proper cabling.

Wireless alarms: Wireless alarms may be used only where the surrounding building construction and environment will not degrade the effective range of the alarm signal. Where a wireless IDS system is used it must meet Federal Communication Commission (FCC) wireless transmission standards.

Environmental Conditions

IDS devices shall be selected and installed to be fully functional under all environmental conditions for the specific location.

Interior Sensors

Interior sensors shall be used to detect the presence of an intruder or an attempt to gain entry into controlled and restricted areas. These areas include, but are not limited to, exterior and interior entrances, such as doors, windows, walls, roof and ceilings, ventilation, underground tunnels and pathways. The following sensor options shall be applied based upon the level of protection required and the type of area to be monitored.

Balanced magnetic switches (BMS): BMS shall be used to detect attempted access or entry of interior and exterior doors and fence gates. BMS may be either recessed or surface mounted; the preferred method is to use a recess mounted switch to reduce the ability to defeat the system.

▸ When double doors or gates require protection, each door shall be fitted with a separate magnetic switch.

▸ Surface mounted switches shall be mounted on the protected side of the door.

▸ When protecting roll-up doors wider than 80 inches, BMS shall be mounted on both left and right sides on the interior side of the door.

Glass break sensors: Sensors shall be used to detect attempts to penetrate glass by detecting vibrations and acoustic emanations associated with breaking or cutting glass. All perimeter windows within 40 feet of ground level and windows accessible from an adjoining building roof or within 25 feet directly or diagonally opposite a window, building, roof or fire escape shall use a glass break sensor. Glass break sensors shall be used on windows that exceed 37 in2 with any dimension greater than eight inches.

▸ Windows with security mesh screen do not require glass break sensors. For windows with air conditioning units installed, the mesh screen must encompass the air conditioner.

Volumetric sensors: Also known as a "space sensor," volumetric sensors shall be used for interior confined spaces. Active or passive sensors may be used. Sensitivity shall be adjustable and set to provide maximum protection while reducing false alarms. PACS shall be provided in protected spaces where volumetric detection is provided and shall activate or deactivate the volumetric sensor upon presentation of a proper access control credential.

Passive infrared sensors (PIR): PIR shall meet the requirements of ANSI/SIA PIR-01, Passive Infrared Motion Detector Stands-Features for Enhancing False Alarm Immunity, and shall be capable of detecting changes in infrared energy or heat. A 360-degree field of view configuration shall be preferred for sensor monitoring purposes, but the final determination of configuration for field of view, which may be 360, 180, 90 or 45 degrees, shall be determined from a field survey and mounting surface availability. Sensitivity of the sensor shall be adjustable to provide the necessary area of protection.

Vibration sensors: The building boundary wall to be protected shall use vibration detection sensors mounted to the wall with close spacing to ensure detection of attempted penetration before the wall is breached. Vibration sensors shall be used in combination with BMS for safes and vaults. Wall mounted shock/vibration sensors shall be provided with LEDs to indicate activation and shall be mounted to provide a clear view of the LED. Except for small areas, sensors zoned together shall not cover more than one wall.

Pressure mats: Pressure mats shall be used on the interior side of an entry way and shall be concealed under a lightweight mat or carpeting. Pressure mats shall be used in conjunction with other sensor technologies and shall not be relied on as the sole intrusion detection device for space protection.

Exterior Sensors: Exterior sensors shall only be used for perimeter protection when the area to be protected is bordered by a fence or physical barrier. Exterior perimeter detection capability shall be applied to fenced areas around a site or building, loading docks, and outside storage areas or enclosures, using volumetric sensors in addition to BMS on access gates. Where CCTV cameras with video motion detection are used, exterior sensors may not be necessary. Facilities that use a fence to define boundaries shall address the use and necessity of fence mounted sensors, microwave sensors or photoelectric beams.

Microwave: Microwave sensors shall use a multiple-beam configuration and only be used when there is a clear line of sight between a transmitter and receiver and the ground is fairly level. Microwave sensors shall not be used near outdoor fluorescent lights.

Infrared system: For outdoor applications active infrared systems shall be used in a multi-beam arrangement to create an invisible fence or corral around the protected area. These systems are affected by fog, rain and snow and shall not be installed where local climatic conditions would cause interference.

Buried cable: For high-risk and mission critical facilities that require perimeter protection or perimeters that do not have a fence that can provide protection, buried cable sensors shall be considered in combination with another outdoor perimeter detection technology. To reduce false alarms, buried cable sensors including seismic, pressure and leaky coaxial cables shall not be used in extreme cold environments where there is heavy ice or locations with heavy ground disturbances, low-flying aircraft, or underground utility lines and pipes.

Fence mounted sensors: Fence mounted sensors include tension wire, capacitance, electric vibration and shock sensors. When using fence mounted sensors, a BMS shall be installed at the pedestrian and vehicle access point gates.

Alarm Conditions

> Conduct a field survey to determine security response capability to all alarm conditions, such as bells, sirens, strobes or silent alarms.

Silent alarms may be integrated with CCTV camera coverage. After activation, the SCC personnel and police shall deactivate and re-set the alarms. You must also decide whether you are going to monitor the alarms (retain proprietary control) or pay a third party to do this (Central Station).

Physical Access Control System (PACS)

The Physical Access Control System (PACS) shall include, but not be limited to: card readers, keypads, biometrics, electromagnetic locks and strikes, and electronic security management system (SMS).

System Elements and Features

PACS devices shall be used for the purpose of controlling access and monitoring building entrances, sensitive areas, mission critical asset areas and alarm conditions from an access control perspective.

This includes maintaining control over defined areas such as site access points, parking lot areas, building perimeter and interior areas that are monitored from a centralized SCC.

System Integration

PACS shall be able to be fully integrated with other security subsystems using direct hardwire or computer interface.

Stand-alone versus Network Multiple-Portal System

Stand-alone: Stand-alone systems shall be used to control access to a single entry control point and shall be available either as one integral unit or as two separate components. Data for the entire user population will be stored within a communication panel for future reference and reporting purposes.

Network multiple-portal system: Multiple-portal systems shall be part of a large network of readers and controllers that are connected to a central processing unit (CPU) that will regulate activities at more than one entry point at a time. All systems will be directly under the control of the CPU and will be programmed to receive periodic programming updates and upload data according to a preprogrammed schedule.

Control/Communications Panel

All panels shall be centrally located within a space that will prevent panels from being damaged, tampered with and accessed by unauthorized personnel.

Electronic Security Management System (SMS): The SMS shall allow the configuration of an enrollment and badging station, alarm monitoring, administrative, asset management, digital video management, intrusion detection, visitor enrollment, remote access level management, and integrated security workstations or any combination of all or some. For instance ID cards can be used for cashless cafeteria systems, gift shops and time and attendance options.

Head-end hardware: Head-end hardware shall provide direct interface of all PACS equipment via a hardwired input.

Entry control software: Software shall allow for programming of the PACS via a CPU. All software shall be updated per manufacturer's instructions.

Network interface devices: Interface devices shall consist of all hardware and software required to allow for full interface with other security subsystems via a CPU.

Records management and reports: The SMS shall have the ability to compose, file, maintain, update and print reports for either individuals or the system.

▸   Individual reports shall consist of an employee's name, office location, phone number or direct extension and normal hours of operation, and shall provide a detailed listing of the employee's daily events in relation to accessing points within a facility.

- System reports shall produce information on a daily/weekly/monthly basis for all events, alarms, and any other activity associated with a system user.
- All reports shall be in a date/time format and all information shall be clearly presented.

Functional requirements: The SMS shall provide the ability to control, program and monitor the PACS and all additional security subsystems that are designed to interface with the PACS and SMS.

Picture ID and Badging Station Interface

The badging station shall provide a form-based interface for the entry of badge holder data and access information. All data, including images, shall be stored on the SMS system server. The badging station shall allow image and signature capture for use in badge production and provide tools for badge design. Both video and digital cameras may be used.

Card Credentials and Readers

All card credentials shall comply with Homeland Security Presidential Directive (HSPD) 12, Policy for a Common Identification Standard for Federal Employees and Contractors, and the Federal Information Processing Standards (FIPS) 201, Personal Identity Verification (PIV) of Federal Employees and Contractors. Smart card implementation shall adhere to the Government Smart Card Interoperability Specification (GSC-IS).

Entry Control Device

All entry control devices shall be hardwired to the PACS main control panel and operated by either a card reader or a biometric device via a relay on the control panel.

Door devices: Entry control devices on a door may be any of the following: electronic strike, electronic mortise lock or electromagnetic lock.

Turnstiles: Turnstiles may be considered as a means of access control as an option to controlling access through lobby areas based on the size and traffic throughput. Depending upon the application, the following security turnstile equipment may be utilized: optical, waist high, drop arm, rotary gate or mass transit.

Biometric Systems

As a means of secondary access control to card readers, biometric devices may be used for high-level control and restricted areas. Biometric systems have unique and limited applications and are not suited to all access control requirements. The types of biometric devices that may be used include hand/palm geometry, fingerprint verification, retinal verification or voice verification.

Portal Control Devices

Portal control devices, such as a push button, request-to-exit or panic/crash bar, shall be used as a means of assisting persons exiting a controlled space and shall provide a secondary means of access control within a secure area. Portal control devices provide the means to override the PACS via a keypad or key bypass and assist in door operations using automatic openers and closures. Portal control devices shall be connected to and monitored by the main PACS panel or SMS.

Door Status Indicators

Door status indicators such as a door position switch or request-to-exit pushbutton shall monitor and report door status to the SMS.

Transmission Media

All PACS control panels shall interface with a CPU in accordance with appropriate media connections. Panels shall be system specific addressable, Internet Protocol (IP) addressable and programmable via a computer. All panels shall be interfaced directly from a computer or via the Internet or Intranet. Access to the panels shall be password protected. All individuals with access to the panels shall be assigned a user specific password.

Think doors, signs and doors locked with keys, then programmable or other cipher locks and/or access systems, and then think biometric.

Duress, Security Phones and Intercom System (DSPI)

The section addresses physical security criteria associated with the selection, application and performance of the intercommunications system, also referred to as duress, security phones or emergency call-boxes, and intercom system (DSPI).

System Elements and Features

The DSPI system is used to provide security intercommunications for access control, emergency assistance and identification of locations where persons under duress request a security response.

DSPI system compatibility: All components of the DSPI shall be fully compatible and shall not require the addition of interface equipment or software upgrades to ensure a fully operational system.

System integration: DSPI shall be fully integrated with other security subsystems.

Handicapped accessibility: DSPI systems shall be handicapped accessible.

Security intercoms: The main components of this security subsystem are the hardwired master intercom and remote intercom stations. Intercom devices shall be integrated with the CCTV system upon initiation and activation of a two-way conversation. Where wireless systems are used, repeaters shall be required. Typical locations for security intercoms shall include:

- Access controlled entry points to a site, parking and perimeter building areas
- Gated access and service road entry points
- Loading docks and shipping/receiving areas
- Interior building access control points to restricted areas
- Exterior building entrances where potential patients will self-report or where there could be confusion as to whether this entrance is a 24-hour entrance or an ED entrance

Intercom door release: Security intercom with remote door release capability shall be used for functional areas that require PACS. The security intercom system shall be integrated with electronic or magnetic remote door release allowing for remote communication and unlocking of doors from a reception desk or SCC master intercom station. The security intercoms for these areas shall have both an audio and built-in video capability. Video verification of person(s) requesting access at these points shall be required.

Intercom master station: The master station shall be capable of selectively calling and communicating with all intercom stations individually or system wide. Master stations shall have a "call in" switch to provide an audible and visual indication of incoming calls from remote stations. The master station shall include, but not be limited to, a handset, microphone/speaker, volume control, push-to-talk button, an incoming call/privacy indicator, and selectors to permit calling and communicating with each remote or other master stations.

Intercom substation: An Intercom substation shall be capable of calling into a pre-programmed single or group of master stations via the pressing of a button or voice activation. When a programmed master station is not available, the call shall automatically transfer to another master station.

Multi-intercom station: The multi-intercom station shall have the ability to call or monitor multiple stations individually or as a public address system.

Single intercom station: A single intercom station only calls or monitors one other intercom location or station at a time; intercoms are direct wired and do not require a master station.

Push-to-Talk (PTT) two-way communications: PTT is the typical type of intercom activation device, which requires that a button is pressed in order to transmit conversation over the intercom.

Voice operated intercom switching (VOX): VOX automatically switches audio direction based on the sound of a voice. The switch works when a sound is detected by the speaker/transmitter and no pushbutton is required to transmit a communication. These intercoms shall be used in interior or exterior areas; however, not in areas with high-background noise such as parking garages.

Security Phones or Emergency Call-Boxes

An emergency call-box or telephone system shall be used instead of intercoms for a multi-facility environment, a stand-alone facility with a parking structure, or a site with a requirement to transmit call station communications to another site. Emergency call-boxes shall be used in areas such as parking garages/lots, sidewalks, pathways of large campuses and in isolated areas. Some intercoms have CCTV capability, as well.

Pushbutton hardwired: Emergency call-box systems shall be hardwired to a master station located and monitored at a central location, preferably the SCC. Pushing and releasing the emergency call-box call button shall initiate a call-in to a pre-programmed master station. Once the button is pushed, hands-free operation shall occur.

Handset-telephone extension: Emergency call-boxes shall have the capability of using the existing PBX telephone system lines. The PBX or CBX shall direct calls to a pre-programmed extension that may be located at a receptionist desk, the SCC, or both. Lifting the handset shall automatically dial a pre-programmed monitoring station. The caller's location shall be defined in the PBX system. A minimum of two numbers shall be programmed into the system, so that if the first number is busy or unavailable the second number will be polled. Facility telephone systems and emergency call-boxes shall not use automatic voice dialers to 911 or the municipal police department.

Speaker-handset stations: Emergency call-box stations shall have the capability to automatically cut out the loudspeaker at the station when the phone handset is lifted, allowing conversations to occur through the handset rather than a speaker.

Scream alert option: Emergency call-boxes shall provide the option that a speaker phone becomes activated when a loud scream is heard. This system shall be limited to indoor applications, such as stairwells and elevators or pre-defined high-threat locations, where background noise will not cause false activation of these devices.

Integration with CCTV Cameras: Emergency call-boxes shall provide coverage with CCTV when activated or have a built-in camera video surveillance capability that can be monitored from the SCC upon device activation.

Remote control and monitoring: Emergency call-box master stations shall have the capability of monitoring and automatically polling each call-box, reporting incoming calls, identifying locations and keeping records of all call events via software and integration with the SMS. The system shall provide auto-answer capability to allow VA Police to monitor and initiate calls. The master stations shall have the capability to remotely adjust speakerphone and microphone capabilities and reset the call-box activation from the central monitoring station.

Signaling devices: Emergency call-boxes shall provide visual recognition devices, such as strobes or beacons, which will provide identification of the activated call-box.

Outdoor vs. indoor locations: All emergency call-boxes shall be installed on rigid structures, columns, walls, poles and/or freestanding pedestals that are easily identifiable through unique markings, striping or paint, signage or lighting, and shall remain easily visible during low-light conditions. CCTV and call-boxes shall be integrated to provide automatic surveillance and priority monitoring of the caller's location.

‣ Emergency call-boxes in indoor locations shall be easily accessible to the public, clearly marked and may be wall mounted.

‣ All emergency call-boxes must be meet handicapped accessibility requirements.

‣ Test frequently.

Duress/Panic Alarms

Duress/panic alarms shall be provided at locations where there is considerable public contact in isolated and pre-identified high-risk areas, such as the lobby reception desk, patient service areas, nursing stations, and isolated offices and buildings where personnel work. Upon activation, a silent alarm signal shall be sent to a centralized monitoring location that shall be capable of continuous operations. Other requirements associated with activated alarms shall include all of the following:

▸ Alarms shall be continuously monitored by the SCC.

▸ Activated alarms shall be integrated with CCTV coverage of the area.

▸ Alarms shall be mounted in such a manner as not to be observable, and shall prevent unintentional operation and false alarms.

▸ At strategic locations use PACS keypads that are capable of activation by a code known only to the user to notify the central monitoring station that the person entering an area is under duress.

▸ Conduct location use risk assessment to determine appropriate locations for installation.

▸ Test every month. Allow a "user" to activate the device. As most are covert, testing is required on a regular basis.

▸ Use anti-false alarm units whenever possible.

Switch/pushbutton hardwired: The duress/panic alarm system shall be hardwired to a monitoring site or the SCC. Upon activation of the alarm, both a visual and audible alarm will be activated in the SCC. The system shall identify the location of the alarm by phone extension and area description.

Wireless: Before selection and installation of a wireless system, a survey shall be conducted to determine if a wireless application is feasible. Wireless systems shall use ultrasonic, infrared and radio frequency waves to link duress/panic devices with distributed transmitters and receivers. Receivers shall be mounted throughout an area or building, as needed, and hardwired to a central monitoring console. Repeaters shall be used to ensure full coverage. All wireless duress systems must conform to Federal Communications Commission (FCC) standards for wireless communications systems.

Switch/pushbutton telephone extension: This system shall use an existing telephone line and PBX to transmit a duress alarm. On activation, the PBX shall direct the signal with the caller's location defined to a pre-programmed extension located at the SCC. Facility telephone systems and emergency call-boxes shall not use automatic voice dialers to 911 or the municipal police department.

Wireless-pendant devices: Wireless duress/panic devices (also known as personal panic alarm, identification duress alarm or man-down alarm) may be considered as an option. When the panic button is pushed a wireless alarm signal is sent to the closest installed wireless sensing unit, which sends the signal on to a designated alarm monitoring location. Only wireless alarms that provide both geographical location and identification of the individual and have been tested in the operational area, especially in isolated areas impacted by structures, topology and other influencing factors, shall be used. The use of these devices shall be limited to personnel identified as holding high-risk positions, work in isolated areas, or travel to/from parking areas and buildings that are isolated, especially during hours of darkness. The devices shall meet the following requirements:

- Be convertible and have the capability to be worn on a lanyard around the neck, belt clip or wristband
- Include rechargeable batteries with low-battery indicators that notify the user and monitoring station of their use
- Be equipped with a pull chain that activates the device should an attempt be made to forcibly remove it from the person carrying it
- Only be operational while on facility property
- Be tested frequently

The duress/panic alarm devices shall be integrated with SCC and SMS software to provide identification and location of the user. Locators shall be required for wireless/pendant devices. Requirements for locators and repeaters shall be as follows:

- Locators shall be placed in strategic locations such as hallways, gathering rooms, parking lots and garages, walking trails or any place where the location of a person in duress is required.
- For large campuses and outside applications, repeaters shall be used that provide true line-of-sight range. The number of repeaters required will depend on the performance of a site survey, capabilities and coverage distances.

Automated dispatch: Duress/panic alarm devices shall automatically announce or provide alarm notification signals to onsite pagers worn by security/police and other designated personnel, hand-held portable radios, cell phones and landline telephones.

Integration with CCTV cameras and Intrusion Detection System (IDS): Duress alarm areas shall be covered by CCTV cameras. Once the duress alarm has been activated, the CCTV system shall monitor and record all events associated with the alarm. The IDS will provide monitoring of duress alarm.

Setting Up the Team

Incident Command

Responsibilities of Incident Command Center (ICC)

The Incident Command Center implements, coordinates and monitors the Emergency Management Plan. (Remember)Specific responsibilities will vary depending on the type and severity of the emergency at hand. This becomes the central communication point during all disasters.

> A common mistake is closing the ICC too soon, and another is overtaxing the staff. Keep shifts to about four hours to ensure staff members stay fresh.

Key Team Members

Any number of titles can assume the job responsibilities for an ICS role. The command center team will include an Incident Commander (who may initially be the nursing supervisor on an off-tour). Other key roles are Administrator on Call, Safety and Security Officer, Public Information Officer; Liaison Officer and Medical/Technical Specialists as needed, down to the Planning, Operations, Logistics and Finance Chiefs. The "three-deep" approach should be practiced in which a designated person and two alternate persons are trained for each key role.

 Remember ————————

The nature of the emergency will also dictate what other team members need to be co-opted. For instance, if there is a terrorist threat, local, state and federal law enforcement will need to be involved.

The HICS organizational structure can be located at: hicscenter.org/docs/163.swf for HICS 203 and Organization Assignment List at www.emsa.ca.gov/HICS/files/hics207.doc for HICS 207 Organization Chart.

Note: NFPA 99 calls for using the same ICS system that the local community uses and NIMS requires that you use HICS.

If there is a major incident or terrorist threat, there may be a need to set up unified command or multi-agency coordination (MAC).

Essential Personnel are those employees designated by Directors/Department Managers as essential for continued operations during an emergency. All management personnel are considered Essential Personnel. Essential Personnel duties are specific to their department's functions and should be defined by each manager in his/her departmental emergency plan.

Teams

Department Directors/Managers may institute Team A (or Alpha)/Team B (Bravo) scheduling as follows:

▸ Team A will remain onsite throughout the initial response phase of an event, and will be released from duty when Team B reports. Delays can occur because of unsafe road conditions including poor visibility, fog, heavy rain, blizzard, ice, flooding, high winds, debris on the roads, or restricted access due to a hostage or terrorist scenario. Staff should be prepared for the possibility of needing to stay at the hospital longer than initially anticipated. This includes having a personal preparedness plan for themselves and their families, and packing a "go-bag" with changes of uniforms, hygiene items and any prescribed medications. In a major disaster or catastrophic event, planning for healthcare workforce relief personnel will need to occur for staffing needs to be sustained.

▸ Team B members will report for duty when directed by the hospital TV or phone hotline message, electronic notification (email, texting) or via direct communication with their Director, Manager or Personnel designee. Team B members are required to remain in contact with their Director/Managers. If unable to reach their Director/Managers, Team B members are required to remain informed by calling the designated call-in system.

Activation of Incident Command Center

The Emergency Operations Plan (EOP) for the hospital details who has the authority to activate the disaster response for the organization. There are a number of titles that can assume the role of the Incident Commander. The plan details the response during normal business hours and for off-tour events. Typically, the nursing supervisor will initially assume the role of Incident Commander during evening and night shifts and on weekends until relieved by the Administrator on-call or HICS designated team response. The plan should incorporate flexibility to scale up or down to the level of response needed.

Incident Command Center (ICC)

The Incident Command Center should be designed to house hospital command personnel in addition to the potential for various state and federal government emergency operations representatives. A primary ICC location and an alternate secondary site should be pre-designated and equipped as follows:

▸ Areas with restricted and controlled access

▸ Minimal to no windows

▸ Positioning away from potential flooding areas

▸ Conference table and chairs

▸ Side office or one in near proximity for conference calls

▸ Air conditioning/heating units

▸ Adequate electrical outlets linked to backup generator power

▸ Dedicated phone lines

▸ Hi-speed Internet access and fax lines

▸ Printer, scanner, copier and television

▸ At least two laptops with installed Intranet/Internet access and additional software to use for internal event management documentation and tracking, and links to external Websites to complete bed availability and other updates to external authorities

▸ Two-way radios to stay in contact with key HICS staff members, as well as a radio to communicate with external contacts

▸ Satellite phone

▸ Spectralink phones

▸ HEAR radio (if needed)

- HAM radio
- External antenna for a ham radio operator; pre-installed cabling will allow for rapid setup
- Whiteboards, easels, paper pads and basic office supplies
- Charging location for emergency radios and cell phones to communicate internally or externally
- A hard and electronic copy of all hospital emergency plans, critical contacts, Memorandums of Agreement with vendors and other hospitals, a staff roster including schedules, and 24/7 contact numbers and home addresses; backup all resources in binders, as well as on a memory stick
- Resource books such as the Federal Emergency Management Agency Field Operations Guide (FOG); Department of Transportation's Emergency Response Guidebook and others that will be helpful for your team
- An HICS roster with designated and alternate staff identified for each key role; Job Action Sheets for each position
- Hard and electronic copies of all ICS forms
- A copy of the hospital campus map, including floor-by-floor blueprints in addition to blueprints for all facilities/buildings affiliated with the hospital
- A map of local area and surrounding communities, floor plan elevations and evacuation routes
- Video and digital camera equipment to document pre-event facility status and post-event damage
- Flashlights, hard hats, personal protective equipment and whistles
- Cots, pillows, blankets and backpacks stocked with basic hygiene supplies
- Water and non-perishable food items
- Refrigerator and coffee pot
- Emergency alert radio (weather)
- HICS position boxes (including vests)
- Television with cable TV and satellite (you could lose cable in a hurricane)
- Battery backup clock

Security

It is important that everyone who needs access to the ICC has photo-ID which must be checked every time they visit the center.

Additional controls might also be needed such as swipe cards or keypad controlled locks to access sensitive areas. The area around the ICC must also be kept secure, and security staff will be required to ensure this with adequate security personnel available around the clock, if necessary.

Developing the Plan

Identifying and Listening to all Internal and External Stakeholders

Because health and medical services include so many different activities, it is essential to establish a framework for these services to work together.

 Tip ──────────────

Consider having a hospital representative sitting in at the ESF 8 desk at the county EOC during any disaster to provide liaison with the county ESFs.

To ensure that the necessary planning and coordination are accomplished prior to the occurrence of a disaster and to facilitate the management of health and medical services during disasters, it is essential to vest this planning and coordination responsibility in one position. An appropriate title for this position is Emergency Management Coordinator or Emergency Preparedness Coordinator. The individual that fills this position is responsible for coordinating EMS, hospital, public health, environmental health, mental health, and mortuary services disaster planning and response actions. The concept of operations should include provisions for:

- Coordinating health and medical response team efforts
- Triage of the injured or ill, as appropriate
- Medical care and transport for the injured
- Identification, transportation and disposition of the deceased
- Holding and treatment areas for the injured
- Isolating, decontaminating, and treating victims of hazardous chemical or infectious diseases, as needed
- Identifying hazardous chemicals or infectious diseases, controlling their spread, and reporting their presence to appropriate state and federal health or environmental authorities
- Communicating public health and medical advisories to hospital staff, medical providers and patients on such matters as emergency water supplies, waste disposal, mass feeding services, vectors, immunizations, disinfection and others.

You can also send a security officer from the closest hospital to the joint command center at the scene to provide onsite intel and also to provide updates from the hospital on census and other information. You will need to meet with your local emergency responders to obtain agreement for this.

In hurricane-prone Brevard County, Florida, special-needs shelters and long-term care facilities are used to prevent filling hospitals pre-storm so that there is capacity post-storm. This allows people with underlying medical conditions to receive attention at a safe location during the storm, including home vent dependent patients.

Organization and Assignment of Responsibilities

Emergency Medical Services (EMS)

▸ Respond to the disaster scene with emergency medical personnel and equipment.

▸ Upon arrival at the scene, assume appropriate role in the ICS. If ICS has not been established, initiate in accordance with the jurisdiction's emergency management system and report implementation to the EOC.

▸ Triage, perform immediate lifesaving interventions, if needed, and transport the injured. Those with emergent needs (red-color disaster triage tags) are treated and transported first from the scene. In a mass casualty incident, stabilization and treatment may not be able to be initially offered beyond lifesaving interventions. A field first aid staging area can be set up to care for minor care casualties, which can reduce the surge on hospitals.

▸ Coordinate casualty distribution to hospitals within the local area or further, if needed, based on the size of the event, level of care needed and bed availability. Take into account criteria to transport casualties to trauma centers and burn centers. Consider the use of clinics to treat minor illnesses and injuries.

▸ Coordinate isolation or decontamination of biological, chemical or radiological casualties, as needed, to decrease exposure and limit dispersion of agents to emergency responders, health and medical providers and treating facilities. EMS should perform gross decontamination at the scene of a contaminated event. Hospitals will follow this up with technical decontamination.

▸ Establish and maintain field communications and coordination with other responding emergency teams (medical, fire, police, public works, etc.), and radio or telephone communications with hospitals, as appropriate.

▸ Direct the activities of private, volunteer and other emergency medical units, and of bystander volunteers as needed.

▸ Evacuate patients from affected hospitals and nursing homes, if necessary.

Hospital Command Team

Upon activation, or upon declaration or imminent declaration of an emergency or disaster:

▸ Reports to the EOC or other designated location as deemed appropriate; sends a representative to the EOC if unable to report in person.

▸ Rapidly assesses health and medical needs.

▸ Oversees and coordinates the activated health and medical organizations to assess their needs, helps them obtain resources and ensures that necessary services are provided.

▸ Coordinates with neighboring community health and medical organizations and with state and federal officials on matters related to assistance from other jurisdictions, including federal assistance.

▸ Verifies valid licensure and proof of identification for health and medical volunteers. Disaster Medical Assistance Teams (DMAT) and Medical Reserve Corps (MRC) volunteers, are pre-registered and pre-credentialed and require only active license verification prior to deployment for missions (in case there have been changes since initial validation).

▸ Maintains a patient tracking system.

▸ Coordinates the location, procurement, screening, and allocation of health and medical supplies and resources, including human resources, required to support health and medical operations (in conjunction with or the responsibility of the Logistics Chief).

▸ The PIO coordinates with the Joint Information Center of the local EOC on the number of injuries and deaths. In a disaster event with distribution of casualties across multiple hospitals, this is the appropriate way to do it.

▸ Ensures appropriate health and medical services information is made available to the information processing section in the EOC.

▸ Coordinates support to the jurisdiction's efforts to respond to inquiries from family members concerned about loved ones.

> Remember: Healthcare is part of the process – it does not drive the process. Hospitals are first receivers, not first responders.

Hospitals

▸ Implement Emergency Operations Plan. The hospital's Comprehensive Emergency Management Plan (CEMP) includes both internal and external responses to hazards. Internal disasters still require communication with external authorities.

▸ Advise the Health and Medical Coordinator or appropriate representative in the EOC of conditions of the hospital and number and type of available beds.

▸ Establish and maintain field and inter-hospital medical communications.

▸ Provide medical guidance as needed to EMS.

▸ Coordinate with other hospitals and with EMS on the evacuation of patients from affected hospitals, if necessary. Evacuation provisions should specify where the patients are to be taken.

▸ Depending on the situation, deploy medical personnel, supplies and equipment to the disaster site(s) or retain them at the hospital for incoming patients.

▸ Establish and staff a reception and support center at each hospital for the relatives and friends of disaster victims who may converge there in search of their loved ones.

▸ Provide patient identification information to the American Red Cross (ARC) upon request.

Note. Patient tracking information may actually be coordinated through ESF-8 Health and Medical at the local EOC versus directly with ARC. You must be aware of HIPAA accountability with protected patient information.

▸ Many dialysis centers may be separate from hospitals and may not have generator backup. They may be offline for some time. Identify a staffing plan to support continued availability of dialysis services for hospital patients.

▸ Many patients may be discharged ahead of a major storm and given prescriptions. Arrangements must be made to provide them with medications, as pharmacies may be closed.

▸ Ensure that hospital and medical staff visibly display their badges while coming to and leaving work and while on duty.

▸ If the hospital is asked by local officials to impose a curfew during the disaster what provisions have been made to provide access to essential staff?

▸ Consider telemedicine triage options from the hospital to the scene.

Note: Consider an employee assistance program, as staff is likely to be impacted by natural disasters. The program could have an emergency roof tarp program, cash advances against pay checks and respite for a few days for employees who have lost homes to give them time to get back on their feet. You must also consider the disposition of staff – where do they live, how might they be impacted by a disaster and how might this impact staffing levels at the hospital. By supporting your staff and taking care of their issues—they can focus on taking care of patients.

The following county officers will also be involved although their focus will be on community issues rather than hospital issues:

Public Health Officer

▸ Coordinates all public health services in the jurisdiction.

▸ Inspects for purity and usability of all foodstuffs, water, drugs and other consumables that were exposed to the hazard.

▸ Provides epidemiological surveillance, case investigating and follow-up.

▸ Provides laboratory services for agent identification required to support emergency health and medical services.

▸ Coordinates operations for immunizations or quarantine procedures, if required.

▸ Establishes preventive health services, including the control of communicable diseases such as influenza.

▸ Monitors food handling and mass feeding sanitation service in emergency facilities, including increased attention to sanitation in commercial feeding and facilities that are used to feed disaster victims.

Environmental Health Officer

▸ Provides for the monitoring and evaluation of environmental health risks or hazards as needed, and ensures the appropriate actions are taken to protect the health and safety of disaster victims, responders and the general public.

▸ Monitors for air-quality hazards and extremes in environmental temperatures.

▸ Implements actions to prevent or control vectors such as flies, mosquitoes and rodents.

▸ Detects and inspects sources of contamination.

▸ Inspects damaged buildings for health hazards.

▸ Coordinates with the water, public works or sanitation departments to ensure the availability of potable water, an effective sewage system and sanitary garbage disposal.

▸ Coordinates with the animal care and control agency to dispose of dead animals.

▸ Ensures that adequate sanitary facilities are provided in emergency shelters and for response personnel.

Mental Health Agencies

▸ Ensure that appropriate mental health services are available for disaster victims, survivors, bystanders, responders and their families, and other community care-givers during response and recovery. Services may include crisis psychological first aid counseling, critical incident stress debriefings, information and referral to other resources, and education about normal, predictable reactions to a disaster experience and how to cope with them. There should be a capacity to provide specialized assistance for those affected by a traumatic event or who become traumatized by cumulative stress related to the disaster experience.

▸ Provide outreach to identify and serve those in need of mental health support.

▸ Coordinate with the JIC to arrange for dissemination of information to the public.

▸ Coordinate with the Mass Care Coordinator to identify shelter occupants that may require assistance.

▸ Have inpatient psychiatric facilities take the following actions:
  ▷ Implement the facility's appropriate disaster plan.
  ▷ Provide for the care, safety and continued treatment of hospital residents.
  ▷ Coordinate with appropriate authorities for the safe evacuation of residents.
  ▷ Provide resources and support to the community-based mental health system in responding to the disaster mental health needs of impacted communities.

Mortuary Services

▸ Provide for the collection, identification and care of human remains, determining the cause of death, inventorying and protecting deceased's personal effects, and locating and notifying the next of kin.

▸ Establish temporary morgue sites.

- Establish and maintain a comprehensive record-keeping system for continuous updating and recording of fatality numbers.

Coordinate with:

- Search and rescue teams, hospitals, EMS and other emergency responders
- Medical Examiners
- Funeral directors, morticians and assets for transportation of deceased persons
- Other pathologists
- The ARC for location and notification of relatives
- Dentists and X-ray technicians for purposes of identification
- Law enforcement agencies for security, property protection and evidence collection

American Red Cross

- Provides food for emergency medical workers, volunteers and patients, if requested.
- Maintains a Disaster Welfare Information (DWI) system in coordination with hospitals, aid stations and field triage units to collect, receive and report information about the status of victims.
- Assists in the notification of the next of kin of the injured and deceased.
- Assists with the reunification of the injured with their families.
- Provides blood, blood substitutes and blood byproducts, and/or implementing reciprocal agreements for replacement of blood items.
- Provides first aid and other related medical support at temporary treatment centers, as requested, and within capability.
- Provides supplementary medical, nursing aid and other health services upon request, and within capability.
- Provides assistance for the special needs of persons with functional or access needs.

Social Service Agencies

- Assist in providing support for vulnerable populations including persons with disabilities, children, the elderly and others.

Animal Care and Control Agency

- Coordinates with veterinarians and animal hospitals to arrange for services for animals, as needed. These might include service, companion or farm animals, wildlife, etc.
- Coordinates with the Environmental Health Officer on the location, collection and disposal of dead animals.

Police and Corrections Departments

▸ Maintains emergency health services at juvenile and adult correctional facilities.

▸ Assists Mortuary Services in the identification of fatalities.

▸ Provides security assistance to medical facilities, and to health and medical field personnel upon request.

Military

▸ Provides personnel and equipment to support medical operations during disaster situations (at the direction of the governor).

Other Tasked Organizations

▸ Adhere to all professional and legal standards in the performance of duties.

▸ Provide ongoing status reports to the ESF-8 Health and Medical representative, including number of deaths, injuries, etc.

▸ Provide and/or receive mutual aid in coordination with the ESF-8 Health and Medical representative.

▸ Provide information to the ESF-8 Health and Medical representative for dissemination of public advisories, as needed.

▸ As needed, coordinate with other emergency health and medical services; with emergency services such as fire, police and public works; and with the ESF-8 Health and Medical representative.

▸ Refer all media requests for information to the ESF-8 Health and Medical representative. Maintain updated resource inventories of emergency medical supplies, equipment and personnel resources, including possible sources of replacements.

▸ Arrange for security to protect vulnerable work sites such as alternate care sites, temporary morgues, etc.

▸ Develop plans to evacuate and/or shelter, as appropriate, patients, staff, equipment, supplies, and vehicles before, during and after disasters. Upload these to Emergency Operations event management Website; review annually at a minimum.

▸ **Prepare detailed SOPs that include:** call-down rosters for notifying personnel; step-by-step procedures for performing assigned tasks; telephone numbers and addresses/locations of similar services in other jurisdictions; area and local stores (grocery and drug), and medical warehouses that will provide pharmaceutical and medical supplies; telephone numbers, addresses, type, quantity, location and procedures for obtaining transportation resources from federal, state, local and private organizations; and a listing of the radio communications call signs and frequencies that each responding organization uses.

▸ Identify designated and alternate staff for disaster roles and responsibilities.

Additional Assets that can be Utilized

Medical Reserve Corps (MRC): You should first identify the chapter leader within the jurisdiction, who has a database of licensed and unlicensed volunteers, to support a health and medical response. Licensed personnel of all healthcare disciplines can enroll in the MRC to support a disaster response with a range of capabilities. All must work under an ESF-8 mission and only within their scope of practice. Students from health and medical disciplines can support a response as MRC volunteers, as long as they are supervised.

Note: MRC volunteers receive training to respond to a disaster. It is not necessary to have trauma/disaster medicine experience. Trauma physicians will most likely be pulled into their trauma centers to support care of the most severely injured. The MRC can support a patient surge with minor care needs, prophylaxis or immunization missions and others. Sketch arrangements for requesting mutual aid teams from neighboring jurisdictions, from state sources, such as state guard or militia units, and from federal sources, such as military, Centers for Disease Control and Prevention (CDC) and National Disaster Medical System (NDMS) sources.

Augmentation Personnel: Identify the sources of other health and medical personnel and the provisions (e.g., verifying adequacy of credentials for those who do not practice in the jurisdiction) that have been made to call upon them to augment disaster medical teams. They include:

▸ Generating a mission request for the local EOC for additional human assets including the capabilities needed. If the local EOC cannot fulfill that request, such as from an MRC pool of volunteers, it will send a mission request up to the state EOC.

Logistics

Sources of medical supplies and equipment:

▸ Local, including hospitals, pharmacies, surgical supply stores, emergency medical services caches, equipment vendors, local government resources, etc. Identify hours of operation for local pharmacies. EMS vehicles have extremely limited inventory; however, most states have EMS caches that are distributed around their states with MCI supplies and pharmaceuticals. Many pharmacies are part of national chains and are private sector entities. They do not have the authority to change their hours with staffing and may not be able to easily receive additional inventory of medications and supplies.

▸ County-stored emergency aid stations, where available and usable.

▸ Mutual aid from jurisdictions not affected by the disaster.

▸ Private sector suppliers in the state.

▸ Private sector health care organizations that maintain a supply system for medical supplies and equipment.

▸ NDMS (includes U.S. Department of Defense, Department of Health and Human Services, Department of Veterans Affairs and FEMA.) **Note:** Local jurisdictions should work through their state emergency management agency and FEMA to obtain resources under the control of the federal government.

▸ Acquisition of medical/health equipment and supplies including:

▹ Initial supply and re-supply for field medical operations

▹ Initial supply and re-supply for health and mortuary services

▹ Re-supply of functioning hospitals in the affected areas

▹ Re-supply of hospitals and other facilities outside the disaster areas receiving casualties

▹ Supply and re-supply of alternate care sites

▸ Transportation of medical/health supplies, personnel and equipment:

▹ Local government-owned and commercial fixed-wing aircraft, trucks and buses

▹ Armed Forces fixed-wing aircraft, helicopters and trucks

▹ Private and public ambulance companies

▹ Water transport

▹ Limousine and taxi companies

▹ Mortuaries (for hearses)

▹ Four-wheel-drive and high-centered vehicles for medical evacuations under bad weather or terrain conditions; Jet skies and/or snow skies

▸ Shelter and feeding of field, health, and medical personnel and patients

▸ Identification and selection of suitable facilities to serve as a temporary morgue

▸ Acquisition of embalming supplies, body bags and necessary heavy equipment suitable for dealing with a mass fatality situation

Plan Development and Maintenance

Hospitals must identify who is responsible for coordinating revisions of the plan, keeping attachments current, and ensuring that SOPs and other necessary implementing documents are developed.

Authorities and References

It is essential that the document contains all statutes, regulations, administrative orders and so on, which provide authority for the preparation of medical and health services disaster plans and for designating the name of the agency and/or title of the officials responsible for management of medical and health services during disaster response and recovery operations.

It should also cite:

▸ Authorities as applicable to coroner/medical examiner and mortuary services during disaster response and recovery operations

▸ Authorities that provide for access to, use of and reimbursement for private sector resources in an emergency and for emergency procurement procedures

▸ Authorities that provide for emergency powers under which emergency medical and public health activities are authorized; also, the extent of liability and/or immunity status of emergency medical, public health and mortuary services workers

▸ References that were used to prepare the jurisdiction's Health and Medical Annex

Communication

Read regional disaster critique reports such as the 2004 hurricane season in Florida, Houston flooding and the Joplin Tornado. Take advantage of best practices and lessons learned to improve your own communication efforts.

Communication during a disaster has at least three equally important components: (1) communication equipment and related systems; (2) relationships and partnerships; and (3) uniform terminology, clearly defined roles and responsibilities, and methods for systematically receiving, fielding and sending communication. During an emergency, communication is a priceless commodity.

☐ Learn from the experiences of others. Share strategies, successes and challenges and obtain knowledge through the lessons learned from other states.

☐ Create a system for managing communication with a goal of reducing excessive calls. NHs need a systematic approach for communicating with emergency management, NH staff, families, regulatory agencies, and suppliers and others during an emergency. If there is not a system in place for managing and fielding communication needs, expect the one phone line that works to be jammed with callers wanting information on everything from available beds to the condition of loved ones.

☐ Be aware of equipment limitations. Satellite phones, though highly recommended, have drawbacks, e.g., limited battery life and transmission failure resulting from excessive and simultaneous queries to one satellite and heavy cloud cover. Text messaging, because it uses less bandwidth and, like email, is not necessarily a "real time" transmission, may be able to get through with minimal delay on an overwhelmed cellular network that has otherwise reached maximum capacity for voice data.

☐ Include ham [amateur radio] operators in communication plans. Ham operators bring their own equipment (receiver and antenna) and operate without the need of satellites or cloudless skies. Licensed by the FCC, ham operators provide backup communication during emergencies worldwide and can be a very dependable communication link when included in a facility's disaster plan. Get to know the ham operator organization serving your area by contacting the National Association for Amateur Radio, (860) 594-0200, or on the Web at www.hello-radio.org/clublist.html. Also consider adding Radio Amateur Civil Emergency Service (RACES) as an organization with local chapters.

☐ Use uniform terminology. When communicating during a disaster, the use of standardized terms and plain language ensures that resources are allocated appropriately. The Department of Health and Human Services (DHHS) has established Hospital Available Beds for Emergencies and Disasters (HAvBED) standards for reporting bed availability specific to various bed types. www.ahrq.gov/prep/havbed/.

Many hospitals are now using event management software to report their bed availabilities, status of their utilities and other key information.

Points to Remember

It is important for Public Information Officer(s) to meet with all external stakeholders on a regular basis to discuss planning and to get to know each other. The first time they meet should not be in the first few hours of a disaster!

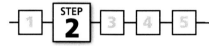

STEP 2
Emergency Specific Responses

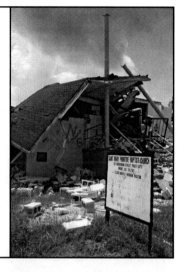

The decision to evacuate is a difficult one. Patients should be evacuated only when absolutely necessary. Situations worthy of evacuation include danger posed by fire, smoke, flooding or a potential exposure to hazardous materials. Evacuation may also be required as a result of facility structural damage or the potential for damage imposed by severe climatic changes, where personnel and patients are in more danger within the facility than any risks posed by evacuation. Not all emergencies will require an emergency evacuation response. The procedures that follow apply only to those situations when an actual evacuation is necessary.

> During any evacuation, unique challenges will be faced due to the physical layout of the facility and the potentially unstable nature of the patients within the facility. All staff members perform important roles in the implementation of an evacuation.

The decision to implement the Emergency Operations Plan (EOP) should be determined by the Incident Commander (according to the facility's HICS model). The Public Information Officer (PIO) is considered part of the Command Center team and reports directly to the Incident Commander. The Incident Commander can initiate activation of notification of an emergency/disaster to the HICS team, and can also initiate mass notification for the facility. The PIO can support the notification process and also provide updates as to the status of an event for hospital staff and media when appropriate. Once a given hospital has activated their plan, a facility's communications department should notify all personnel involved.

When an incident occurs in a clinical area that requires emergency evacuation, hospital personnel assume the responsibility to move patients in immediate danger and also to activate the hospital's emergency code. This will augment assistance to relocate patients and, through the activation of the HICS, coordinate the response for a partial or full evacuation of the facility, as needed. The objective is to get patients and personnel to safe areas of refuge.

Hospital employees should immediately assume the responsibilities of their assigned roles upon activation of the EOP. Hospitals maintain memorandums of agreement with other hospitals with the same level of care. The Hospital's Command Center can activate those agreements and coordinate inter-facility patient transfers. If a hospital is in a disaster status, the city's local Emergency Operations Center and the county or region's EOC will be notified, as well. Ambulance transports (often via a non-emergency ambulance provider) will be prioritized for critical care patients and for patients who are non-ambulatory. Assistance with securing alternate transport vehicles can be accomplished for patients who are ambulatory if there are insufficient ambulance vehicles as would be anticipated in a catastrophic-level event. Other alternatives must be established before an event so you need MOSs with other providers such as bus companies, local airlines and so on.

When the decision is made to activate the EP, the magnitude of the emergency response must be determined. For large-scale events or total facility evacuation, the Liaison Officer (or the Incident Commander) should immediately notify the Office of Emergency Management and other local agencies to establish, as needed, inner and outer perimeters. Emergency Medical Services need to be notified, as well as other hospitals, to determine how many beds are available and the types of patients that can be accepted. If, for instance, a regional evacuation is taking place because of an imminent threat from a Category 5 hurricane or after a F5 tornado hit, then state, regional and federal agencies may need to be involved.

If your city or region is facing, or has just undergone, an imminent catastrophic event, it is likely that first responders and law enforcement will be stretched to the limit, so this must be taken into account when planning for large-scale regional-wide evacuations.

 Must Do ───────────

You must practice large-scale region-wide evacuation drills, whether as tabletop exercises or otherwise, to ensure they work. This should be done at least once every year.

Evacuation of health and medical facilities, shelters and community staging sites will need to be coordinated with the local EOC. Agreements with other hospitals should be established, for example DASH I, DASH II or VHA. It is also important to plan transportation assets which are usually limited, especially in the middle of the night. One Florida hospital lost power and then lost its generator because it couldn't replace a $12 part. As a result, the hospital had to be evacuated.

Bomb/Terrorism

All bomb threats have to be taken seriously and emergency planning must contain contingencies and procedures for such eventualities.

Bomb Threat Procedures:

▸ Use a Bomb Threat Checklist when a threat is made.

▸ Alert the employees. Each facility will determine its own internal alerting/warning procedures. Hospitals use a designated emergency code for a bomb threat and have a standard operating guideline for such an incident. Setting off the fire alarm may be an inappropriate action.

▸ Call 911 and report the threat.

▸ Notify the facility administrator.

▸ Notify facility security personnel.

Evacuation:

No Action

If the bomb threat has been evaluated to be a hoax or a prank, normal operations shall continue.

Partial Evacuation

Depending upon the location, size and nature of the suspect bomb or explosive agent, a partial or full evacuation will be recommended by local law enforcement. A partial evacuation order includes the immediate vicinity of the suspect bomb including areas above and below. The exact distance for evacuation will be estimated by law enforcement subject-matter experts. Note: ATF has recently updated their chart for evacuation distances depending on the type of explosive. One rule of thumb for suspected bomb threats is 500 feet in every direction. In a small hospital, unfortunately, this might mean a large section of the hospital. This would be difficult to do, however, if it turns out to be just a threat. Always bear in mind that patient evacuation may not be readily available.

Complete Evacuation

To signal a complete evacuation, an appropriate overhead emergency code announcement will be ordered. Using emergency codes is intended to alert just staff and not to alarm patients, visitors and others.

Fire doors can be closed to offer additional containment protection.

In patient areas, follow Evacuation Plan guidelines.

In non-patient areas, employees shall:

▸ unlock desk drawers, lockers and file cabinets

▸ turn off equipment and machinery, as appropriate

▸ remove all purses, briefcases, personal packages and lunch boxes (reducing amount of objects that need to be searched)

Supervisors shall confidently assist and direct evacuees, providing reassurance as needed.

Evacuees and unauthorized personnel shall not be allowed to reenter any area during an evacuation.

Facilities Management shall prepare to shut off any reactive building utilities. Services which could add to the force of the explosion, such as gas and fuel oil, shall be shut off in most cases.

Do not use any electronic devices (cell phones, spectrolinks, etc.) until the incident has been cleared.

It is recommended that you evacuate the building to a safe area outside (500 feet from the bomb's most probable location). It is important that the call taker attempts to learn the bomb's approximate location within the facility or adjoining structure(s) during the threatening call.

- Keep all evacuees and employees together in the safe area and wait until first responders arrive. Remember that in the Atlantic abortion clinic bombing, a second device was deliberately positioned to cause additional casualties as people fled the scene from the first. Never assume that there is only one explosive device.

- The threat CALL TAKER should be available to talk to first-arriving response units and provide all available information concerning the call to fire department and law enforcement personnel.

- Law enforcement will monitor the situation from the command center and will decide what action to take.

- Do not re-enter the facility until told it is safe to do so by law enforcement personnel.

Bomb Search By Employees:

- As you evacuate your work area (if that is possible), look for suspicious object(s)/package(s) that do not belong there.

- For those unable to leave, it is important to have life safety drawings available and to drill with the local bomb squad.

- The results of employees searches should be reported to the command center who should ensure that all areas have been searched.

- REMEMBER that there might be more than one bomb, i.e., as in the Atlanta abortion clinic bombing.

- DO NOT touch or attempt to move any strange object/package.

- It is not necessary to move furniture, books or open desk drawers. A visual work area search should take no more than five seconds as you leave your work area.

- Look HIGH, look LOW and ALL IN BETWEEN. Floor to hip, hip to shoulder, shoulder to ceiling.

- As you are exiting the facility, visually scan the hallways and open doorways for strange object(s)/package(s) or anything out of the ordinary.

- Report any suspicious object(s) and/or packages(s) to the hospital command center, and they will report to the appropriate fire department and law enforcement personnel who will respond.

- Make sure someone is assigned to check locked areas and common areas.

> The U.S. Postal Service Website has a number of good resources on this at http://about.usps.com/publications/pub166/pub166fm_012.htm

When conducting a room search, follow the following procedures to ensure a systematic combing of the entire area.

☐ During all searches, two-way radios and cell phones shall remain turned off.

☐ After entering the room, listen for peculiar sounds. Look for objects that appear to "not fit in" with the immediate setting.

☐ Search in a clockwise direction and use a grid search process.

☐ Search the entire floor first.

☐ Search the entire room at both knee and waist levels, opening drawers and cabinets.

☐ Search areas at the head and overhead levels.

☐ If a suspicious package is encountered, DO NOT TOUCH IT! Close off the area, and do not let anyone re-enter until authorities arrive.

☐ Immediately report the location and description to security, other search team members in the area and the Emergency Management Group.

Employees search areas, and the law enforcement officer assigned to this call will most likely go directly to the command center.

Re-Entering The Facility After Being Cleared

Normally law enforcement or the fire department will give permission for staff to re-enter, but some hospitals take this decision themselves if the facility has been searched and nothing found.

▸ Be alert, visually scan the areas again. DO NOT take a bomb threat lightly. Remember that hospitals may have to take special precautions, such as sandbagging the device, if evacuation of patients is not an option, i.e. they are in the ICU or on the operating table.

Post-Detonation/Explosion:

▸ Check employees and residents/patients for injuries.

▸ Call 911 if the call has not already been made or the device detonates/explodes before or immediately after the caller hangs up. This then usually becomes a Code Red response.

▸ Administrator will ensure relatives of employees and residents/patients are notified, as necessary.

▸ The role of the PIO is very important in this phase.

Note: Large facilities may want to expand on the accompanying Bomb Threat Checklist because the call taker would probably be able to attempt to keep the caller on the line a while longer, while other employees carried out Bomb Threat Preparedness duties. You are encouraged to contact your local Police or Sheriff's Department for assistance in expanding on the checklist. Small facilities are expected to pay attention to the minimum checklist items in the hope of being able to help law enforcement officials identify the caller.

If your phone lines are recorded, quickly make a recording for law enforcement.

Telephone Bomb Threat Checklist

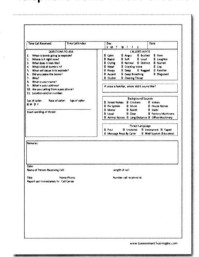

Blank Forms are available online. Please see Table of Contents for instructions.

Ask the Police or Sheriff's Department for assistance in expanding on the checklist. Small facilities are expected to pay attention to the minimum checklist items in the hope of being able to help law enforcement officials identify the caller.

Bomb Threat Caller – Checklist

Blank Forms are available online. Please see Table of Contents for instructions.

Information contained in this checklist can be very helpful to law enforcement personnel in identifying, apprehending and prosecuting the caller. It is recommended that this checklist be started while the caller is still on the line. Finish filling out the checklist as soon as possible after the caller hangs up the phone. Make and keep several copies of this checklist or the checklist you develop. Place a copy next to each business phone. It is also useful to have a copy of the responses to various emergencies posted in every unit and department.

Exercises: This annex will be exercised at least once per calendar year. Exercises are expected to be Homeland Security Exercise and Evaluation Program (HSEEP) compliant which means that there are goals and objectives for the exercise, pre-assigned evaluators (preferably external), an after-action review and a corrective action plan (with specific performance measures to be improved, with dates of anticipated interventions and who is assigned the responsibility. Some hospitals conduct one drill a year as part of their ASPR grant using HSEEP.

The next exercise should reevaluate that there is performance improvement based on recommended corrective actions. HSEEP info can be found on the Web at: hseep.dhs.gov/pages/1001_HSEEP7.aspx.

Documentation of the annual exercise, as determined by your HVA, will include:

☐ Date of the exercise

☐ List the type of exercise: BOMB THREAT

☐ Results of the exercise: Satisfactory: YES _____ NO _____ (Satisfactory indicates that each procedure listed was accomplished safely and in a timely manner.)

A "NO" checkmark indicates one or more of the procedures was not accomplished safely and/or in a timely manner. You should write a very brief description of the problem and the action(s) taken to correct the deficiency. It is recommended that you re-accomplish the portion(s) or the exercise that was unsatisfactory to ensure the revised procedure(s) will work. A suggested "Bomb Threat Procedures Exercise Record" sheet follows.

Bomb Threat Exercise Record

Blank Forms are available online. Please see Table of Contents for instructions.

Bio-Terrorism

These would include the need for medical/technical experts including the Hospital's Infection Control Practitioners (now known as Infection Preventionists), county and state public health and epidemiologists, FBI, state laboratory personnel, law enforcement, CDC, public health department and veterinarians. A biological incident can result in a patient surge that is insidious. Patients initially come in slowly and then the numbers can surge exponentially. There is also a fear factor with an unknown biological agent. This will reflect itself in patients presenting thinking they were possibly exposed but are without symptomatology, healthcare workforce anxieties and possibly call-outs, and staff illness, among others.

> ▶ **Remember** ——————————
>
> Hospitals would be among the first institutions affected after deployment of a weapon of mass destruction. There are measures that would need to be taken for a bioterrorism event.

Patients exposed to biological agents may occasionally also need decontamination, such as for the anthrax incidents in 2001 with weaponized anthrax. Also containment measures will be critical to limit person-to-person spread. Isolation and quarantine interventions may also be needed.

After a biological attack, emergency departments might be the first to note changes in the epidemiology of an infectious disease, to initiate a public health department referral to identify the causative organism and to treat patients affected by the exposure. After a biological, chemical or radiological attack, patients may require decontamination at the hospital if they are contaminated and have bypassed the emergency medical service scene decontamination stations.

> Eighty percent of patients will self-report to a hospital for a multiple casualty incident (MCI).

The number is probably even higher after a contamination event with few people willing to wait until the fire department can set up decontamination centers.

After an explosion, large numbers of injured patients might be brought to emergency departments for treatment. The most seriously injured will be brought in by the emergency services, but, by then, the emergency department might well be full with less seriously injured people who headed straight for the hospital. Internal surge planning is necessary for these situations.

In any of these scenarios, hospitals would experience an influx of patients who may have been exposed and have medical or psychological issues to be addressed. The previous information does not take into account psychological casualties, usually a ratio of 4:1 - about four times more than those physically injured although this can vary depending on the nature of the incident. When there was a radiological leak in Brazil, the ratio was 400:1 – a reason why you need internal surge plans.

Because of the heavy demand placed on their services at the time of an attack, hospitals need to be prepared to handle the workload. And, because the most common terrorist attacks to date have been explosive or incendiary (car bombs, airplanes full of fuel, etc.), hospitals must be prepared to treat an influx of trauma cases. Hospitals must also be prepared to diagnose and treat diseases caused by CDC Class A bioterrorism agents (smallpox, anthrax, plague, botulism, tularemia and hemorrhagic fever). Although hospitals are required to have disaster response plans to be accredited by The Joint Commission (TJC), the standard elements of these plans are still quite general regarding terrorism.

The key to rapid intervention and prevention is to maintain a high level of vigilance. To minimize the number of casualties, early identification that an outbreak is from an unnatural source is essential. A bioterrorist event may be suspected when increasing numbers of otherwise healthy persons with similar symptoms seek treatment in hospital emergency departments, physicians' offices, or clinics over a period of several hours, days or weeks. The early clinical symptoms of infection for most bioterrorism agents may be similar to common diseases seen by health care professionals every day. The principles of epidemiology should be used to assess whether each patient's symptoms are typical of an endemic disease (influenza) currently circulating in the community or an unusual event. The most common features of an outbreak caused by bioterrorist agents include:

- A rapid increase (hours to days) in the number of previously healthy persons with similar symptoms seeking medical treatment

- A cluster of previously healthy persons with similar symptoms who live, work or recreate in a common geographical area

- An unusual clinical presentation

- An increase in reports of dead animals

- Lower incidence rates in those persons who are protected (e.g., confined to home; no exposure to large crowds)

- An increase number of patients who expire within 72 hours after admission to the hospital

- Any person with a history of recent (within the past two-four weeks) travel to a foreign country who presents with symptoms of high fever, rigors, delirium, rash (not characteristic of measles or chick pox), extreme myalgias, prostration, shock, diffuse hemorrhagic lesions or petechiae; and/or extreme dehydration due to vomiting or diarrhea with or without blood loss

Role of the Infection Control Practitioner

The hospital infection control practitioner (ICP) will play a significant role in the rapid identification of an outbreak of community-acquired infection and the notification of local health departments. The ICP is responsible for managing the day-to-day activities of the hospital-wide infection surveillance, prevention and control program. Because the role is highly visible in the hospital and surveillance for infections is a primary function, the ICP is in a unique position to detect rapid or subtle increases in patients admitted with unusual clinical presentations, increases in emergency room visits and Intensive Care Units (ICUs) admissions.

Advising staff of an alert and the case definition of a specific threat will help to identify potential suspect cases as early as possible.

 Must Do

Heightened surveillance in the emergency department and for admitted patients, especially those in critical care units, is vital to the early recognition of a bioterrorism event.

The medical record of all new patients admitted with unusual infectious disease symptoms that go undiagnosed for more then 48 hours should be reviewed. The ICP should, at a minimum, review several times each week all admission diagnoses, microbiology reports and emergency room admission and discharge diagnoses. The emergency department and CCU should communicate any unusual infectious disease patterns to the ICP as soon as possible. It is essential that the ICP develop a clinical syndrome monitoring system for those departments that are likely to be the first affected by a bioterrorism event, such as the emergency department. A clinical syndrome monitoring system could include a method of alerting the ICP when a threshold of the following events is exceeded:

- Increased ED visits, increased critical care admissions, increased overall admission rate, increased admitted patient holding rate or ED diversion status

- Increase in the number of persons with sepsis or septic shock
- Increase in the number of patients with influenza-like illness (ILI); fever, rash, acute respiratory symptoms or infection, acute gastrointestinal distress (nausea, vomiting and/or diarrhea), acute neurological infection, hemorrhagic illness, sudden onset of shock, coma or death, or acute symptoms consistent with botulism
- Increase in the number of patients going the same location with similar symptoms
- Increase in the number of persons with sudden onset of illness who give a history of being otherwise healthy
- Unexplained deaths occurring in otherwise healthy persons, especially if there is clinical evidence suggestive of an infectious disease process

Training and Education

Hospital employees should receive basic information during orientation about the hospital's emergency codes, disaster plan, protective measures, personal preparedness, their roles and responsibilities within their department, and how the Hospital Incident Command System will be activated within the context of a community response.

Subsequent training can build on that foundation with CBRNE training (chemical, biological, radiological, nuclear and explosive), correct donning and doffing of personal protective equipment, use of respiratory protection and other awareness, operational level and specialty courses.

Drills and exercises should be conducted periodically to assess the level of staff preparation. Hospitals should participate in city, county and/or state bioterrorist drills as these events are scheduled. The hospital bioterrorism response plan should be evaluated and revised annually, based on the results of internal and external drills and, as agent updates, detection and treatment information becomes available. Infection control practitioners should be well informed of and participate in state and local bioterrorism preparedness planning and exercises.

Decontamination of Patients and Environment

In most cases, patient decontamination will not be necessary. The incubation period of biological agents makes it unlikely that victims of a bioterrorist event will present immediately following the exposure event. The one exception may be an announced release of a bioterrorist agent, with gross surface contamination of victims with a confirmed agent or material such as raw sewage. In the rare cases where decontamination may be warranted, simple washing with soap and water is sufficient. If necessary, environmental surfaces can be decontaminated with a U.S. Environmental Protection Agency (EPA) registered sporicidal disinfectant or with a 0.5 percent hypochlorite solution (one part household bleach added to nine parts water). Bleach solution should NOT be used to decontaminate patients or pets.

Note: While it is true that most of the CDC Category A agents have a significant incubation period, there are other more common illnesses, such as norovirus, that are not related to a bioterrorist event, but have a fairly rapid spread. Biological illness tends to present with an insidious onset. Patient presentations can start off slowly, one person at a time, and then increase exponentially until the facility feels stressed from the demand. Because staff members are busy taking care of the incoming, it is critical that leadership recognize the increased presentations and activate their surge plan and HICS, as needed, for a scalable response.

Evidence Collection

In some cases, the FBI or other law enforcement agency may require collection of exposed clothing and other potential evidence.

The hospital ICP can guide staff in the collection of lab specimens per guidance from the state Department of Health or per the Centers for Disease Control (CDC). If bioterrorism is suspected, the hospital's vacuum tube system should not be used to transport specimens. Instead they need to be hand-carried and lab staff notified to take additional precautions handling such specimens. There are training programs available for lab staff in packing and shipping of specimens to advanced capacity labs. Local law enforcement can help hospitals develop Standard Operating Guidelines (SOGs) for evidence collection. Chain of custody must be followed with evidence collection and storage.

The FBI field office may follow-up on concerns for bioterrorism; however, it is usually local law enforcement that becomes initially involved.

 Remember ────────────

The primary goal in any bioterrorist event is protecting public safety, and all else is secondary.

By the time the first patients seek treatment and a bioterrorist event is suspected, there may be no evidence to collect. However, hospitals do need to prepare for the possibility that they may be responsible for evidence collection, and there should be policies and procedures in place to collect patient's clothing and other personal effects. In the event that the bioterrorist event is announced, it will become even more important that an orderly procedure is in place for the collection of evidence.

In collaboration with local law enforcement and regional FBI representatives, hospitals should establish lines of authority about who will be responsible for evidence collection. Procedures should include how weapons brought in by patients (e.g., guns, knives and syringes) will be retrieved, secured and handed over to law enforcement officials.

At a minimum, hospitals should have a supply of paper and plastic bags, marking pens, labels and tape to secure the bags. Paper is recommended to protect DNA evidence and to put on hands of deceased persons who may have gunshot residue. Tape is preferred as chain of custody transfer can be recorded across the tape surface (to show that the package has not been opened since evidence was collected). Many hospitals ask persons to be decontaminated to put their clothing in a plastic bag with a bar coded identifier (usually part of a patient Decon Kit). In an MCI, often these plastic bags are stored together in a barrel initially during the decon process.

Each individual bag should be labeled with the patient's name, medical record number, and date and time of collection. Forms should be developed to inventory valuables and provide documentation of the person responsible for the valuables. If valuables are to be transported to the FBI or local law enforcement agency, the facility should document who received them, where they were taken and how the valuables will be returned to the owner.

During routine valuables collection, hospitals use valuables envelopes to inventory items and they are secured with a copy of the envelope number given to the patient with instructions for how to retrieve their items. However, if it a terrorism event and there is significant contamination, valuables may not be able to be returned to people.

Preparing for a Large Influx of Patients

No hospital is ever fully prepared for a sudden large influx of patients requiring critical life support systems. This is the primary reason why hospitals should be represented in local and county emergency preparedness planning. Decisions will have to be made as to whether one hospital in the city or county will be designated as a bioterrorist hospital or if all hospitals will share equally in the influx of patients. When the number of patients exceeds the number of available beds and staffing, decisions will have to be made as to whether alternative care sites will be opened, who will staff these facilities, and how to they will be supplied and re-supplied. This poses a dilemma because hospital staff will be needed at the hospital, so who will staff the alternative case sites? Does the public even know where these sites are, and do they have faith in them?

Many hospitals have agreements with local DOH nurses that during a major mass casualty incident they respond to the closest hospital and become green station nurses. These agreements should be reviewed at least annually to update competencies and complete primary source verification of licensing.

At the hospital level, major decisions will have to be made and implemented quickly. Some of these decisions will include:

- Implementing the hospital emergency operations plan and bioterrorism response plan
- Canceling non-emergency surgeries and other elective procedures
- Discharging patients who can safely go home or to a lower level of care (Reason: When a hospital is in surge mode, census reduction is a good strategy to increase capacity for an anticipated surge of incoming patients.)
- Discharging patients to other acute-care facilities out of the affected geographical area, or to long-term care or home care and ensuring that the level of care required by these patients can be met
- Increasing stock supplies of personal protective equipment (In the event of an incident, such as the H1NI outbreak every available respirator is snapped up rapidly with none available to late comers.)

- Increasing stock supplies of antibiotics and other needed pharmaceuticals
- Determining the availability and sources of additional medical equipment such as ventilators and IV pumps, and other equipment normally rented
- Deciding when it is safe to discharge patients with communicable diseases and developing specific discharge instructions including recommendations for caregiver protection, hand washing; disinfection of the environment and post-mortem care
- Reviewing mass fatality management plans which include surge measures for the morgue

Hospital Tiers

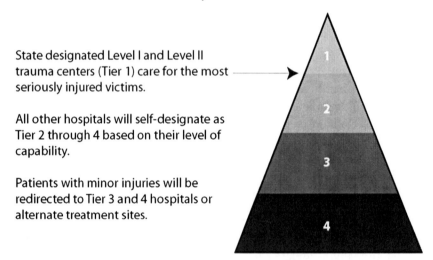

State designated Level I and Level II trauma centers (Tier 1) care for the most seriously injured victims.

All other hospitals will self-designate as Tier 2 through 4 based on their level of capability.

Patients with minor injuries will be redirected to Tier 3 and 4 hospitals or alternate treatment sites.

Injury Severity

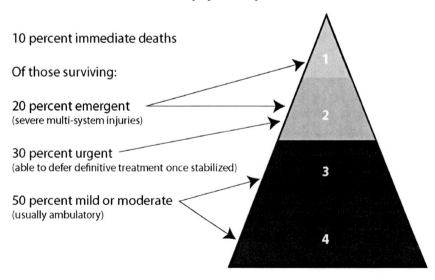

10 percent immediate deaths

Of those surviving:

20 percent emergent
(severe multi-system injuries)

30 percent urgent
(able to defer definitive treatment once stabilized)

50 percent mild or moderate
(usually ambulatory)

Patient Decontamination

Hospitals now maintain Emergency Response Teams which pull from services that can readily support a response. ED, Security, Maintenance/Facilities and Environmental Services need to support a response; however, the team can comprise diverse staff backgrounds. The approach now is to have an alpha-bravo decon team that has a team number appropriate for the size of the hospital and capable of responding to an event – including a surge of patients requiring decontamination.

The need for decontamination depends on the suspected exposure, and in most cases – other than biological - will not be necessary. The goal of decontamination after potential exposure to a bioterrorism agent is to reduce the extent of external contamination of the patient and contain the contamination to prevent further spread. The decision for decontamination should be initiated in the case of gross contamination and in consultation with local Hazmat EMS, hospital medical/technical specialists, and local or state health departments.

 Tip —————————————————

Special provisions must also be made for decontaminating small children and babies.

In the absence of agent-specific guidance, exposed areas should be cleansed using a copious amount of plain soap and water. Potentially contaminated clothing should be removed as soon as practical by staff. However, coordination of this function with outside agencies, i.e., FBI field office or other law enforcement agencies may be necessary, since they may require the collection of exposed clothing and other potential evidence for submission to CDC, FBI or Department of Defense laboratories to assist in exposure investigations.

Health First, which operates four coastal not-for-profit hospitals in Brevard County, Florida, has developed "doff and don" kits so, while waiting for a shower, individuals can remove clothing (doff) and, after showering, there are kits for donning a Tyvek suit. The kits have instructions in English and Spanish and contain other items, such as a small soap bar, moist towelette, and so on.

Doff and Don Kit Contents

Blank Forms are available online. Please see Table of Contents for instructions.

Managing the Psychological Aspects of Bioterrorism

Following a bioterrorism event, anxiety and alarm can be expected from infected patients, their families, health care workers, and those who are fearful or distressed.

Psychological responses may include anger, fear, panic, unrealistic concerns about infection, fear of contagion, and paranoia and social isolation. Infection control practitioners should include mental health workers (psychiatrists, psychologists, social workers and clergy) when developing facility-specific bioterrorism response plans. The following are some points to consider:

▸ Communicate clear, concise information about the infection, how it is transmitted, what treatment and preventive options are currently available, when prophylactic antibiotics, antitoxin serum or vaccines will be available, and how prophylaxis will be distributed.

▸ Provide counseling to those who are fearful or distressed, including support for family members of casualties.

▸ Provide educational materials in the form of frequently asked questions.

▸ Provide home care instructions.

▸ Provide information on isolation and quarantine (isolation is the intervention more likely to be initiated first. Quarantine measures are complex to support and less likely to be used.).

▸ Information released to the public should be coordinated through the Joint Information Centers of local and state EOCs with input by local, state or federal health officials.

The Media

The media should be informed about bioterrorism and the potential disease agents. Following the identification of a bioterrorist event, the local or state health department should assume responsibility for coordinating information to the media through the Joint Information Center of the local or state EOC. Hospitals can provide updates as to their number of casualties and symptoms to their ESF-8 representative. The total casualty number from all hospitals who have received patients can be released as an aggregate through the JIC. In addition, the JIC can release fact sheets about the agent involved including symptoms, preventive measures that can be taken, treatment and treatment locations.

Laboratory Support

With the possible exception of Yersinia pestis (plague) and some food- or water-borne disease agents, most hospital clinical laboratories are not equipped to identify bioterrorist pathogens. These laboratories will primarily be responsible for collection, packaging and transportation of specimens to the county or state laboratories. Each clinical laboratory should develop specific policies and procedures for collection, packaging and transporting specimens to the next level of expertise. Infection control practitioners should consult with local law enforcement and the FBI to determine what information should be included in chain-of-custody documents. Laboratories collecting blood specimens for serology testing should retain an aliquot for a short time to accommodate lost specimens. The retained blood specimens should be kept in a secure, locked cabinet.

During a bioterrorist event, laboratory personnel should take maximum precautions when handling specimens. Laboratory personnel should wear appropriate personal protective equipment when handling all clinical specimens, and all specimens should be opened, plated or aliquotted in a biosafety hood.

The Pharmacy

The pharmacy should maintain a reasonable, daily inventory of antibiotics currently recommended in the treatment of patients with suspected or diagnosed bacterial bioterrorist agents. The CDC has made significant progress in building emergency stockpiles of antibiotics, as well as other emergency medical supplies (intravenous therapy supplies and other emergency medications), that can be available within 12 hours after the federal government confirms that a bioterrorist event is in progress. Hospitals should develop criteria for stopping the non-essential use of prophylactic and therapeutic antibiotics until the stockpile arrives at the local destination and preparations are made to distribute the stockpile resources. Hospitals must also plan for events, such as an approaching hurricane, when businesses including pharmacies close. However, you still have patients being discharged with scripts and also from the ED post-storm when the pharmacies have not yet re-opened.

Discharge Planning

In all probability, patients in the hospital at the time that a bioterrorist event is evolving will have to be evaluated for quick discharge. If patients require continued acute care, hospitals may have to make arrangements for transfers to other hospitals or, if stable, to skilled nursing facilities in different geographical areas. Patients with bioterrorist-related infections should not be discharged until they are deemed non-infectious (plague, smallpox and viral hemorrhagic fever).

These instructions were developed primarily for caring for patients who could not be admitted to the hospital because maximum bed capacity and staffing levels had been reached or exceeded. These instructions can be modified to provide information for patients recuperating from an infectious disease. Most bioterrorist agents are rendered non-infectious by exposure to air and sun. Therefore, no specific recommendations for packaging and removing medical waste from the home are necessary. However, the ICP should consult with local waste management companies and the local or state government medical waste program for recommendations related to removing regulated medical wastes from the home.

Post-mortem Care

Hospitals should assess the maximum number of deceased persons that can be stored in the facility morgue at any one time. In the event that many people expire within a short period, hospitals should plan for temporary morgue surge space and coordinate planning with their local emergency operations center and medical examiner office to provide transportation, refrigeration and disposition of diseased persons.

Hospitals should use their routine process to support identification of patients. The Medical Examiner's office has the expertise to assist with those who remain unidentified.

Standard Precautions

Standard Precautions, as defined by the Centers for Disease Control and Prevention (CDC), are designed to reduce the risk of transmission of most disease causing microorganisms in any type of health care setting regardless of the patient's presumed or diagnosed infectious status. With the exception of smallpox, viral hemorrhagic fevers and pneumonic plague, most infectious diseases caused by bioterrorism agents are rarely, if ever, transmitted from person-to-person. Standard Precautions should be integrated into all health care worker/patient care interactions that include contact with:

▸   Blood

▸   Non-intact skin

▸   Body fluids, regardless of the presence or absence of visible blood (urine, feces, vomitus, wound and lesion drainage, pulmonary secretions including nasal and salivary secretions and tears)

▸   Skin soiled with visible blood or other body fluids

▸   Mucous membranes

Health care workers should follow facility specific policies and procedures related to reducing the risk of occupational exposure to blood and other potentially infectious materials, as required by the Occupational Safety and Health Administration's Blood-borne Pathogens Standard. Place patients in any available bed on any nursing unit. Patients with similar syndromes may also be cohorted (grouped) in semi-private or multiple-bed rooms. Special ventilation may or may not be required. Consider placing patients who frequently contaminate the immediate environment with blood or body fluids (e.g., incontinence, wound drainage not contained by a dressing or poor hygienic habits) in a private room.

Limit visitors to immediate family members and significant others. Instruct visitors to wash their hands before and after patient contact and before leaving the patient's room. In a major incident, hospitals might have to completely restrict visitors.

The use of personal protective equipment (PPE) – gloves, respiratory protection, goggles (eye protection) or face shields (respiratory and eye protection) and gowns, as well as hand washing are essential requirements. See OSHA standards to determine whether you are in class 1, 2 or 3.

Fire Safety

Since smoking has been "eliminated" in many hospitals, the majority of fires in health care are now in the kitchens, according to NFPA, so specific attention to kitchen fires and training is required. This should include discussing the K type fire extinguisher. TJC published a Sentinel Event Alert on surgical fires a few years back for ambulatory centers. While rare, the possibility of such incidents must be addressed, as the impact is significant.

1. **Minor Fire Actions and Evacuation Procedures:** defined as a minor fire as one that is not structural in nature, i.e., fire in a trash can. It is strongly suggested that you contact the local fire department that would respond to a fire at your facility and work together in determining what size fire, type of fire and location of fire would constitute a minor fire. A small skillet or saucepan fire can be extinguished by shutting off the heat source and covering the skillet/pan or by using common table salt. A dry powder fire extinguisher is also effective but very messy.

    ▷ When a fire is detected or smoke from an unknown source is detected, activate pull station fire alarm.

    ▷ Evaluate the need for horizontal evacuation.

    ▷ If safe to do so, close all interior doors and look for the fire location as you evacuate – as appropriate.

    ▷ Perform a head count to ensure all persons are out of the building.

    ▷ Notify 911 and report your problem for assistance in checking the building for safety purposes.

    ▷ Notify the Administrator if not on the property.

    ▷ Make sure someone is designated to turn off medical gas/oxygen zone valves.

    ▷ Remember that TJC requires a minimum number of fire drills and each has to be evaluated as a "pass" or "no pass."

Note: Many facilities still have fire blankets – especially in lab and plant operations area - but the NFPA reports that when people wrap themselves in fire blankets, the flames are forced up to the head and face. According to the ECRI, fire blankets should never be used in surgical fire settings. A risk assessment should be completed, keeping this in mind and whether fire blankets are right for your facility.

> It is a good idea to indicate to staff where smoke compartments start or end. Signs can be placed on door frames stating, for instance, "Smoke Compartment door." This is done to inform the staff, not patients.

2. **Major Fire Actions And Evacuation Procedures:** A major fire usually involves the structure or a portion of the structure. It could also be a deep-fat fryer fire or similar appliance if it is burning out of control. Another major fire source would be (if applicable to the facility) the natural gas line at the side of a facility. If the line is broken, there is always the possibility of ignition. If the facility uses a 500 or 1,000 gallon propane gas tank for heating and/or cooling, there is a potential for leaks, fire and even an explosion. Contact the local fire department that would be the first response unit and ask for assistance in determining your facility's potential vulnerability to a major fire.

   ▷ Activate pull station alarm

   ▷ Begin evacuating all persons from the building. Some campuses have multiple buildings, and you can evacuate beyond a two-hour separation.

   ▷ If safe to do so, close all interior doors and look for the fire location as you evacuate.

Note: Hospitals have fire doors that will automatically close if there is a fire alarm pulled. Interior doors of patient rooms will also need to be closed once cleared that there is no threat in each room. If patients are evacuated from the rooms, signal that the room has been cleared and checked with the designated method for the hospital. This can be through use of tape across the door, an X mark on the door or through tags hung on the door handle to indicate a cleared room.

   ▷ Perform a head count to ensure all persons are out of the building.

   ▷ Do not re-enter the building.

   ▷ Go to the nearest building that has a phone, and ask someone there to call 911.

   ▷ Assign staff to remain with evacuated patients to attend to their needs.

3. **Fighting The Fire:** Firefighting priorities in order are, protect human life, protect private property and protect the environment. Hospitals use the acronym RACE: Rescue patients in immediate danger; Sound the Alarm; Contain the fire (close the door of the evacuated room with the fire) and Extinguish the fire using a fire extinguisher if possible. Initially only patients in immediate danger are moved from the area. Others are moved as needed if the fire is not contained and extinguished. Your local fire department's safety representative is your best source of information and planning assistance. Remember, a MINOR FIRE can become a MAJOR FIRE very quickly.

   ▷ If it is a small incipient fire, tackle it straight away or have the hospital fire response team handle it.

4. **Evacuation Procedures:** Every hospital has their own evacuation route to a pre-designated staging area.

For LTC facilities, list each area of your facility, including utility room(s) and common area bathrooms and indicate the primary and secondary evacuation routes out of the facility. If your facility is a multi-level (two stories or more; don't forget the basement area) do the same in-depth planning.

5. **Exercises:** This annex will be exercised at least once per calendar year. Documentation of the annual exercise will include:

   ▷ Date of the exercise: Must be exercised once per year, any time.

   ▷ List the type of fire exercise (MAJOR or MINOR).

   ▷ Results of the exercise: Satisfactory: YES _____ NO _____ (Satisfactory indicates that each procedure listed was accomplished safely and in a timely manner.)

A "NO" checkmark indicates one or more of the procedures was not accomplished safely and/or in a timely manner. You should write a very brief description of the problem and the action(s) taken to correct the deficiency. It is recommended that you re-accomplish the portion(s) or the exercise that was unsatisfactory to ensure the revised procedure(s) will work.

NFPA stipulates what is required for a fire drill. In addition, you should consider issues such as patients in restraints, forensic patients and how long it took the central station to call 911. Consider the impact that sprinklers will have on the fire.

A suggested "Fire Procedures Exercise Record" sheet follows.

Fire Procedures Exercise Record

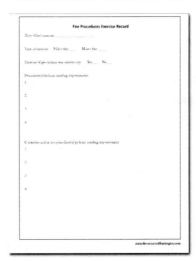

Blank Forms are available online. Please see Table of Contents for instructions.

Extreme Weather

An earthquake in Washington DC and a tropical storm that caused massive flooding in the northeast - both once in a lifetime events - illustrate why emergency planning has to take into account the impact of extreme weather.

Severe Cold Weather Procedures:

Under normal circumstances the facility's heating unit(s) will provide a comfortable environment. The following steps should be taken when/if the facility's heating unit(s) become inoperative.

▸ Notify the appropriate heating repair personnel.

▸ If the heating repair company indicates an unusual amount of time to repair the unit, evacuation can occur to one of more other hospitals as bed availability and patient acceptance by receiving MDs occurs. Hospitals should maintain MOUs with other hospitals with same levels of care, in case they need to serve as a host receiving facility or the one that needs to evacuate.

▸ If you decide to move to another facility, notify your Local Emergency Management Office for coordination purposes.

▸ If an evacuation of a nursing home is necessary, the Administrator will ensure family members are notified.

▸ Keep persons dressed warmly.

▸ Get blankets ready for use in case they are needed.

▸ Provide warm liquids for residents.

▸ If electrical power is interrupted for more than five (5) minutes, notify the Administrator.

▸ Indicate how you intend to provide and prepare food for your residents.

Severe Hot Weather Procedures:

Hospitals have generators and even backup generators, so there is usually minimum interruption to power. Under normal circumstances the facility's cooling unit(s) will provide a comfortable environment. The following steps should be taken when/if a nursing home or assisted living facility's cooling unit(s) becomes inoperative, and there is no backup generator.

▸ Notify the appropriate air conditioning repair personnel.

▸ If the air conditioning repair company indicates an unusual amount of time to repair the unit, consider relocating to a paired facility.

▸ If you decide to move to another facility, notify your Local Emergency Management Office for coordination purposes.

▸ If an evacuation of the facility is necessary, the Administrator will ensure family members are notified.

▸ If a person appears to be in any danger of heat-related stress, call 911.

▸ Provide cool liquids for persons to drink.

▸   Use fans to circulate air.

▸   Provide cold wash cloths as needed.

▸   If electrical power is interrupted for more than five (5) minutes, notify the Administrator.

▸   Indicate how you intend to provide and prepare food for your residents.

Exercises: This annex will be exercised at least once per calendar year. Documentation of the annual exercise will include:

▸   Date of the exercise: Severe Weather HOT exercise must be accomplished prior to MAY each year. COLD Weather exercise must be accomplished prior to NOVEMBER each year.

▸   List the type of severe weather hot/cold exercise (HOT or COLD):

▸   Results of the exercise: Satisfactory: YES _____   NO _____ (Satisfactory indicates that each Procedure listed above was accomplished safely and in a timely manner.)

A "NO" check mark indicates one or more of the above procedures was not accomplished safely and/or in a timely manner. You should write a very brief description of the problem and the action(s) taken to correct the deficiency. It is recommended that you re-accomplish the portion(s) or the exercise that was unsatisfactory to ensure the revised procedure(s) will work. A suggested "Severe Weather Hot/Cold Procedures Exercise Record" sheet follows.

Severe Weather Hot/Cold Procedures Exercise Record

Blank Forms are available online. Please see Table of Contents for instructions.

Severe Storms

Hurricane Katrina was one of the worst natural disasters in U.S. history. Some inpatient facilities, including hospitals and nursing homes, evacuated due to the hurricane. Some facilities evacuated before the storm, while others evacuated after the storm because they were unable to sustain operations.

Storms, Tornadoes and Hurricanes

When a **Severe Thunderstorm Watch** is issued for your area:

▸ Notify the Administrator and staff that a Severe Thunderstorm Warning has been issued for your area and include timeframe of warning. Larger facilities may have a designated position to perform this function. Some hospitals allow the call center operator to call a Code Purple once a "warning" has been sent out and tornados are sighted or are presumed based on local radar.

▸ Begin monitoring the storm system on radio, TV or National Oceanographic Atmospheric Administration (NOAA) Weather Alert Radio.

▸ Have a battery-powered portable radio available to backup commercial and auxiliary electrical power systems.

When a **Severe Thunderstorm Warning** is issued for your area:

▸ Notify the Administrator and staff that a Severe Thunderstorm Warning has been issued for your area and include timeframe of warning. (Larger facilities may have a designated position to perform this function.)

▸ Begin monitoring the storm system on radio, TV or National Oceanographic Atmospheric Administration (NOAA) Weather Alert Radio.

▸ Have a battery-powered portable radio available to backup commercial and auxiliary electrical power systems.

▸ Close all exterior doors and windows.

▸ Keep all persons away from windows.

▸ Close cubical curtains, and move patients away from windows.

▸ Ready pillows and blankets so if weather worsens, you are prepared.

▸ If any injuries are sustained by staff members or residents/patients, call 911.

▸ In case of injury to residents or if residents/patients experience other medical problems, the Administrator will be responsible for ensuring family members of injured or ill residents/patients are notified as soon as possible.

▸ If there is any damage to the facility and/or surrounding area, your Local Emergency Management Director will provide you with the department and number to call.)

Add one or more bullets to the preceding list that states how you will provide emergency food and water for your residents/patients. Your Local Emergency Management Director can provide you with some helpful pre-disaster tips regarding emergency food, water and other essential supplies.

Hurricane Watch – A watch is announced when hurricane conditions are possible within 36 hours for a particular area.

Hurricane Warning – A warning that sustained winds 64kt (74mph or 119km/h) or higher associated with a hurricane are expected in a specified coastal area in 24 hours or less. A hurricane warning can remain in effect when dangerously high water or a combination of dangerously high water and exceptionally high waves continue, even though winds may be less than hurricane force.

The Saffir-Simpson Hurricane Scale is a 1-5 rating system used to define a hurricane's intensity. It gives an estimate of the potential property damage and flooding expected along the coast from a hurricane landfall. Wind speed is the determining factor in the scale, as storm surge values are highly dependent on the slope of the continental shelf and the shape of the coastline in the landfall region.

> Note that all winds are defined using the U.S. National Weather Service's definition of sustained winds which is the average winds over a period of one minute.

Category 1 Hurricane – Winds 74-95 mph (64-82 kt). Storm surge is generally four-five feet above normal. No real damage to building structures. Expect damage primarily to unanchored mobile homes, shrubbery and trees and some damage to poorly constructed signs. Also, expect some coastal road flooding and minor pier damage.

▸ **Examples:** Gaston 2004, Lili 2002, Irene 1999 and Allison 1995.

Category 2 Hurricane – Winds 96-110 mph (83-95 kt). Storm surge is generally six-eight feet above normal. Expect some roofing material, door and window damage of buildings and considerable damage to shrubbery and trees with some trees blown down. Considerable damage to mobile homes, poorly constructed signs and piers. Coastal and low-lying escape routes flood two-four hours before arrival of the hurricane center. Small craft in unprotected anchorages break moorings.

▸ **Examples:** Frances 2004, Isabel 2003, Bonnie 1998, Georges 1998 and Gloria 1985.

Category 3 Hurricane – Winds 111-130 mph (96-113 kt). Storm surge is generally nine-12 feet above normal. Expect some structural damage to small residences and utility buildings with a minor amount of power failures, and damage to shrubbery and trees with foliage blown off trees and large trees blown down. Mobile homes and poorly constructed signs are destroyed. Low-lying escape routes are cut by rising water three-five hours before arrival of the center of the hurricane. Flooding near the coast destroys smaller structures with larger structures damaged by battering from floating debris. Terrain, continuously lower than five feet above mean sea level, may flood inland up to eight miles (13 km) or more. Evacuation of low-lying residences within several blocks of the shoreline may be required.

▸ **Examples:** Katrina 2005, Jeanne 2004 and Ivan 2004.

Category 4 Hurricane – Winds 131 – 155 mph (114-135 kt). Storm surge is generally 13-18 feet above normal. Expect more extensive power failures, damage to doors and windows with some complete roof structure failures on small residences. Shrubs, trees and all signs are blown down.

Complete destruction of mobile homes. Low-lying escape routes may be cut by rising water three-five hours before arrival of the center of the hurricane. Expect major damage to lower floors of structures near the shore. Terrain that is lower than 10 feet above sea level may be flooded, requiring massive evacuation of residential areas as far inland as six miles (10 km).

▸ **Examples:** Dennis 2005 (Cuba) and Charley 2004.

Category 5 Hurricane – Winds 156 mph and up (135+ kt). Storm surge is generally greater than 18 feet above normal. Expect complete roof failure on many residences and industrial buildings and other complete building failures with small utility buildings blown over or away. All shrubs, trees and signs may be blown down. Complete destruction of mobile homes. Expect severe and extensive window and door damage. Low-lying escape routes are cut by rising water three-five hours before arrival of the center of the hurricane. Major damage to lower floors of all structures located less than 15 feet above sea level and within 500 yards of the shoreline. Massive evacuation of residential areas on low ground within five-10 miles (8-16 km) of the shoreline may be required.

▸ **Examples:** The Labor Day Hurricane of 1935, Hurricane Camille (1969) and Hurricane Andrew (1992).

The 1935 Labor Day Hurricane struck the Florida Keys with a minimum pressure of 892 mb – the lowest pressure ever observed in the United States. Hurricane Camille struck the Mississippi Gulf Coast causing a 25-foot storm surge.

Evacuation Decisions

A pre-event evacuation may be carried out in anticipation of an impending event, when the hospital structure and surrounding environment have not yet been compromised. A pre-event evacuation is appropriate when decision teams believe the effects of the impending disaster may either place patients and staff at unacceptable risk, or when an evacuation after the event is likely to be extremely dangerous or impossible.

Pre-event evacuations are an option in Advanced Warning Events – disasters that decision teams and emergency officials can anticipate and track, as they assess the possible consequences of the disaster on their hospital and the surrounding community. Hurricanes are the most common example of Advanced Warning Events, and decision teams may decide to evacuate prior to hurricane landfall. If decision teams elect not to preemptively evacuate, deciding instead to shelter-in-place, a post-event evacuation may become necessary, depending on the impact of the event on the hospital and surrounding area.

Figure 1. Advanced Warning Event Evacuation Decisions

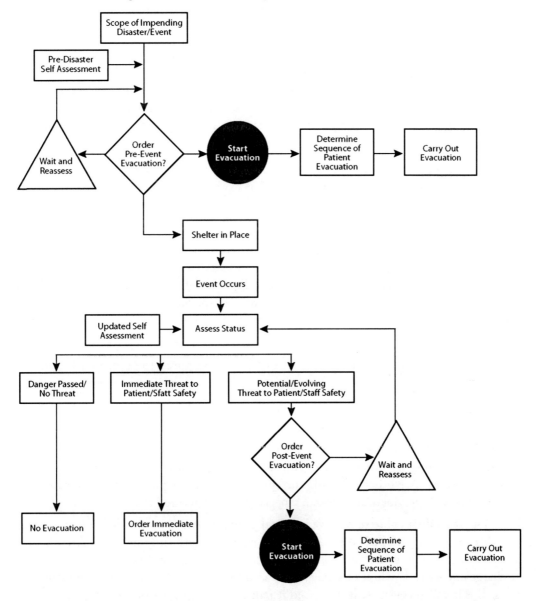

There are several possible "paths" through the Figure 1 flowchart, including ordering a pre-event evacuation following a wait and reassess period; deciding to shelter in place, with no subsequent evacuation required; and deciding to shelter in place following a wait and reassess period, and then subsequently ordering a post-event evacuation.

The flowchart begins with an initial consideration of the decision to order a pre-event evacuation. Typically, this would occur as soon as a disaster is identified that could potentially threaten a hospital. This is often days before the disaster "hits," such as when a hospital is inside a three-day projected hurricane path. The flowchart highlights the three possible outcomes of this decision: wait and reassess, start an evacuation or make an explicit decision to shelter in place during the event.

The wait-and-reassess option defers the decision of whether to start a pre-event evacuation and is typically the preferred option early in the tracking period, when the disaster is not yet an immediate threat. The wait-and-reassess option is predicated on the decision teams' belief that after reassessment, there will still be ample time remaining for an evacuation, if it is needed. In this option, disaster tracking meetings are held regularly, and decision teams cycle through the flowchart loop of "Order Pre-Event Evacuation" and "Wait and Reassess" possibly several times.

Decision teams rely on emergency management officials for accurate information about both the expected time and magnitude of the event, as well as explicit quantification of the uncertainty of estimates. Of course in some situations, such as a verified bomb threat, there may be no time to "wait and reassess."

In the wait-and-reassess option, the expected time until the event occurs should be compared to the time required to evacuate patients from the building and safely transport them to other facilities to determine if the decision to evacuate can be deferred. The evacuation time assumptions generated as part of the Pre-Disaster Self-Assessment provide estimates for the time required to safely evacuate. These assumptions should be revisited based on current conditions in the hospital and the expected impact of the event.

Specific items to consider in the reassessment of the time required to evacuate patients include the following:

▸ **Current patient census and mix.** How does the current patient census differ from the assumptions used to estimate evacuation time and resource needs in the self-assessment?

▸ **Availability of ambulances, wheelchair vans and buses.** Are previous assumptions about the availability of transportation resources still valid? Are alternative sources of transportation resources available? Are other hospitals currently evacuating or planning to evacuate patients? Agreements with providers are needed, especially if patients are being moved out of county.

▸ **Location of facilities able to receive hospital patients.** Are the intended receiving care sites still able to accept patients? What alternative receiving care sites are available to accept patients? When there is time, particularly in the days prior to a hurricane, decision teams usually discharge any patients who can safely be released to their families and stop admitting elective cases. This is called census reduction, and it reduces the demands on the hospital as the focus turns to evacuating patients who require ongoing care. Census reduction may take place before an official pre-event evacuation order is given, as in advance of hurricane; early discharges may also occur after a No Advanced Warning Event, such as an earthquake. Census reduction is a deliberate strategy to reduce the number of patients a hospital is responsible for transferring to other facilities.

▸ **Pre-Event Evacuation or Shelter in Place?** The wait-and-reassess option is viable for only a limited period of time; as the event progresses and conditions deteriorate, patients will not be able to be evacuated safely due to, for example, hurricane-force winds or impassable roads. At some point, decision teams must decide whether to evacuate the hospital or shelter in place during the event. Hospitals prefer shelter in place rather than to evacuate.

What Hospitals Can Expect: Pre-Storm

> It is important to align your plan with the local EOC.

96 - 72 Hours in Advance. During this time, there is much uncertainty regarding the path and intensity of a storm. This is a good time to review plans, implement just-in-time training and finalize staffing plans. Notifications and communication plans and systems should be tested and implemented and emergency operation centers may be partially activated. Since hurricanes may expand over large areas and their paths are uncertain, it is likely that all hospitals in the state will need to prepare to implement their hurricane plans. For those hospitals that may need to evacuate, this is the time to assess the potential situations and begin making evacuation decisions.

72 - 48 Hours in Advance. During this time, there may still be some uncertainty, but there will be a better sense of what is to be expected. Hurricane response plans should be activated and final preparations made. Supplies need to be secured and staff assignments need to be confirmed. Staff and the community should be implementing their personal and family preparedness plans. Buildings and homes will be boarded up and sandbags may be filled and appropriately placed. You can expect crowded roadways and stores due to people gathering supplies. Evacuations may begin during this time. The Emergency Operations Center may be fully operational and holding briefings on a frequent basis.

36 Hours in Advance. Final preparations are being made, evacuations have begun and supplies and resources are being staged. Response plans should be activated, including Incident Command. Briefings with multiple stakeholders will be occurring. For example, you may have regularly scheduled briefings with the Emergency Operation Center (EOC), the state and other hospitals/hospital association. Planning meetings may become more frequent. Additional communication devices may be distributed at this time. Unmet just-in-time training needs should be addressed. Consider canceling elective procedures.

24 Hours in Advance. At this time, all of your preparedness plans should be activated and implemented. Any unmet needs should be addressed. Staff (and family) that will be staying at the hospital during the storm will be arriving. Keep in mind storm conditions set in before the actual landfall of the eye of the hurricane. You need to make sure that staff is at the hospital prior to the onset of storm conditions. Community shelters should be open, and residents will be traveling to check into the shelters. Storms may stall, change course or increase/decrease in intensity prior to landfall. Once you have activated your response plan and everything is in place, there may be a period of time where you are simply waiting for the storm to hit. Incidents of panic may exist as stress builds from the waiting.

What Hospitals Can Expect: Post-Storm

First 24 Hours Post-Event. Once severe weather has subsided, and it is daylight, you can begin assessing the damage to your facility, and the status of staff and resources. Search and rescue operations may be conducted in your surrounding communities, and community damage/impact assessments may also be underway. Facility and partner incident management teams should already be in full operation. Staff will be anxious to connect with loved ones and to know the status of their homes.

During this time consider the following:

▸ Conduct impact assessment and prioritize needs. It is during this time that evacuation decisions may be made contingent on operational capacity. If you are not evacuating and operating at a severely diminished capacity, you also may need to consider requesting additional resources such as a Disaster Medical Assistance Team (DMAT) and/or Medical Reserve Corps support.

▸ FEMA damage assessment teams – important if you want some financial support.

▸ Staffing pre- during and post-storm.

▸ Special needs consolidation plan.

▸ Dialysis patients.

▸ Patients that ran out of home oxygen.

▸ Begin hurricane planning in January.

▸ Contract with employees.

▸ Child care for pre- and post-storm.

▸ Create a booklet summarizing your plan.

▸ Exemption criteria for not working during storm.

▸ Department checklists (IT does not want you to unplug the network connection just the power).

▸ Pre-hires video that spells out role and responsibility that health care staff are expected to be there during an emergency event including hurricanes.

▸ Pets.

▸ Staffing special needs shelters.

▸ Seat at EOC – ESF 8 desk (health and medical).

▸ Sandbags.

▸ Respite maps for in-house support of staff.

▸ Water supplies.

- ▸ Generator support.

- ▸ DMAT support? Where?

- ▸ Executive staffing.

- ▸ Identify additional resources needed and make requests accordingly.

- ▸ Assess status and need to activate continuity of operations plan (COOP). Has it been activated? Are any areas of your facility experiencing or are going to experience diminished capacity due to the effects of the severe weather event? Hospitals may need to activate COOP in appropriate units of hospital during recovery operations.

- ▸ Remove debris. When planning for recovery, consider pre-staging resources such as front loaders, salt and sand. Ensure vendor contracts are in place to promptly remove debris and/or snow promptly following an event.

Health First had an all or nothing plan and changed it to allow for modifications as no two situations are the same. F or example Tropical Storm Faye dropped more than 28 inches of rain in Cocoa Beach and, while it was not a wind event, staff couldn't get to work. While the average speed of a moving hurricane is 12 mph – Hurricane Faye moved at an average of five mph while Hurricane Charley moved at 25 mph across the Florida peninsula.

24 – 48 Hours Post-Event. Depending on the severity of the event and the amount of time it takes to clear roads for safe travels, staff should be able to be rotated during this time. Hospitals need to be prepared to assist staff with the hardship they may face from damaged homes, and the closures of schools and childcare centers. Community resources and activities are most likely still discontinued, placing additional burden on hospitals to meet the needs of the community and staff.

During this time period, a patient surge may be noted from people tending to damaged homes, being involved in motor vehicle crashes if intersection lights are out and other mechanisms of injury. In addition, if there is significant damage to the community, security may need to be increased to address the influx of persons seeking shelter, food, air conditioning/heat and other basic human needs.

 Tip ━━━━━━━━━━━━━━━

Hospitals, however, should work with their human resource departments to advance cash from their next paycheck to staff needing it.

The hurricane planning, response and recovery toolkit provides information on examples of staff support. For example, if banks are closed and it is pay day, can you pay staff in cash? Will you provide administrative leave to staff needing to take time off from work to meet with insurance claims processors? Will you loan funds to employees to help them pay upfront high-deductible costs? Many hospitals have a bank branch at their facility; however, this service is unlikely to be on generator power (that also includes the ATM service).

48–72 Hours Post-Event. Hospitals should plan for the worst and still be able to be self-sufficient during this time. What to expect during this time can vary significantly, depending on the severity of the event and the state of community resources. If there is significant damage to community infrastructure, including widespread power outages and damage to homes making them not habitable, you will continue to have delays with patient discharges, most likely be operating on generator power, begin running low on supplies and the media may be present with continued inquiries on the status of your facility's operations. In addition, if dialysis centers are not operational, dialysis patients will begin seeking treatment at hospitals. For less severe events, demobilization and scaling back or standing down the incident command team may begin.

72 Hours Post-Event. If the event is severe enough and demobilization has not yet occurred, there will be a need to continue to manage issues but perhaps at a higher level of intensity. Fuel will be in high demand by all, not just for facility generators but also for transportation for staff. Generator use in the community also leads to concerns of carbon-monoxide poisoning. Generators may have been running long enough that maintenance tasks will need to be performed (i.e. change filters, change/add oil). Staff may be growing weary, and, if schools are still closed, childcare/elder care for family members of staff will continue to be a concern. Emotional and mental health support will need to be provided to health care workers and family members in the coming days and months. Hospitals need to plan to be self-sufficient for 96 hours or implement evacuation plans.

Hospitals Closely Monitor Track of Hurricane Rita

The University of Texas Medical Branch (UTMB) initiated its hurricane preparedness procedures on Sunday, September 18, 2005, five days prior to landfall of what was then Tropical Storm Rita. When Rita was officially classified as a hurricane on Monday and was headed towards UTMB's location on the upper Texas coast, the medical center initiated census reduction efforts to discharge as many ambulatory patients as possible. On Tuesday, three days prior to landfall, the incident command center opened in accordance with UTMB's emergency operations plan. All unit-level emergency plans were also activated, bio-safety level three and four labs were closed and decontaminated, and medical students and nonessential personnel were dismissed. Late Tuesday evening, a teleconference was held between UTMB and the Texas Department of Public Safety's Division of Emergency Management, during which the Department guaranteed UTMB adequate ground and air transportation for a full evacuation, if the evacuation decision was made by 7:00 the following morning. From Tuesday evening until the time of the final decision on Wednesday, UTMB assessed and triaged patients, copied medical records, assembled patient medication lists and contacted a large hospital network to determine the number of transfers they could accept. At 7:00 a.m. Wednesday, two days prior to landfall of Hurricane Rita, a hospital-wide evacuation was ordered.

Take a look at the location of Cape Canaveral Hospital (www.health-first.org) which sits on a spit of land in the middle of a river and one mile from the Atlantic Ocean. Every east to west storm with a direct impact forces an evacuation which is why Health First probably has more evacuation experience than anyone else. That is why they developed a Web-based program for evacuation which also allows other hospitals to monitor the patients they are being sent. It is also another reason why evacuation drills are practiced regularly. In 2004, the hospital was evacuated twice in just over a two-week period.

Cape Canaveral Hospital

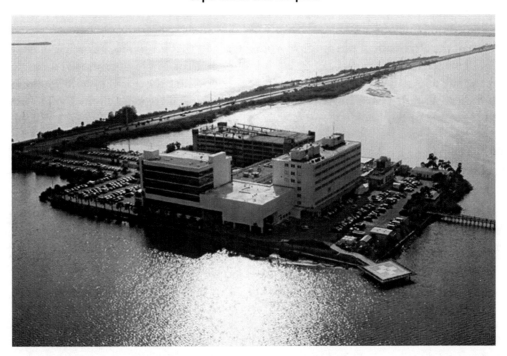

Deciding whether to preemptively evacuate or shelter-in-place requires consideration of two factors:

▸ The nature of the event, including its expected arrival time, magnitude, area of impact and duration; and

▸ The anticipated effects on both the hospital and the community, given the nature of the event and the results of the Pre-Disaster Self-Assessment.

Decision teams will, of course, closely monitor impending disasters in order to gauge anticipated effects on the hospital and the surrounding area. Four generic disaster characteristics to be monitored include: arrival time, magnitude, geographic area affected and duration. Perhaps more important than the estimate of these characteristics is the variability around that estimate and how likely the variability could potentially change. The most common example of variability is the width of the hurricane "cone" showing the projected path of the hurricane.

Local emergency management and other experts are the best source of information on event characteristics. At a minimum, hospital decision teams should educate themselves on disaster-specific characteristics, their variability, and what factors affect variability. For example, movement of wildfires is affected by three main factors: weather, fuel (e.g., ground material) and topography. In the case of river flooding, the areas that will be flooded at varying flood stages – in particular, the key roads to a hospital – should be documented and included in hospital evacuation plans.

Tornadoes

The images of the aftermath of the multiple-vortex tornado that hit Joplin, Missouri, in May 2011, show how devastating these events can be. Winds of more than 200 mph destroyed more than one third of the city and claimed 160 lives. Emergency services and the population of Joplin had just 24 minutes' lead-in time before impact. A report on the medical response to the Joplin Tornado is attached at the end of this book.

Tornado Watch:

▸ Notify the Administrator and staff that a Tornado Watch has been issued for your area and include timeframe of warning.

▸ Begin monitoring the storm system on radio, TV or National Oceanographic Atmospheric Administration (NOAA) Weather Alert Radio.

▸ Have a battery powered portable radio available to backup commercial and auxiliary electrical power systems.

▸ Be prepared to transition from a Tornado Watch to a Tornado Warning with little or no advance warning.

Tornado Warning:

▸ Notify the Administrator and staff that a Tornado Warning has been issued for your area and include timeframe of warning. Some Florida hospitals allow their call center operators to enact their Code Purple process to minimize delays in a response.

▸ Close all exterior doors and windows.

  ▹ Close all interior doors.

  ▹ Ensure all staff members and residents are moved to the interior hallways and have a pillow and blanket.

▸ If your facility has a basement, move everyone to the basement instead of hallways.

▸ Staff members and residents will remain at their Tornado Warning shelter area until the warning has expired and/or the storm cloud has passed.

After The Tornado/Winds Have Passed:

▸ Check staff members and residents/patients for injuries.

▸ Check the facility and immediate outside area for damages.

A. **Electricity** – Does the facility have electrical power? Look for downed power lines, trees on lines and/or storm debris on power lines.

B. **Water** – Does water flow when faucets are turned ON? Is the water color normal? Does it have an unusual odor?

C. **Gas (if applicable)** – Does gas appliances work when turned ON? Is a there an odor of gas (rotten eggs)? Are gas lines/regulators outside the facility intact?

▹ If your facility has a residential propane storage tank, is it still upright? Is the fuel supply line from the tank to your facility intact? If you suspect a leak or hear a high pressure, hissing or whistling sound release in progress, move everyone upwind and uphill from the leak and extinguish or guard against potential ignition sources.

D. Look at damage to the facility and use your judgment as to whether or not it is safe to occupy the facility. If you determine the building is unsafe for occupancy, notify the Local Emergency Management Agency by calling _____. (The Local Emergency Management Office will provide you with the number to call.)

E. If an evacuation of the facility is necessary, patients and staff will move to an alternate pre-designated location. The Administrator will ensure family members of the patients are notified as soon as possible concerning any medical problems, injuries and/or evacuation of the facility.

> Prior to moving patients, you should coordinate with the local EOC ESF-8 contact.

Exercises: This annex will be exercised at least once per calendar year. Exercises as a general rule, need to be addressed via the HVA and will focus on the most likely scenarios based upon impact, frequency, duration and so on. Documentation of the annual exercise will include:

▸ Date of the exercise: Must be accomplished each year.

▸ List the type of severe weather exercise (THUNDERSTORM or TORNADO).

▸ Results of the exercise: Satisfactory: YES _____ NO _____ (Satisfactory indicates that each Procedure listed above was accomplished safely and in a timely manner.)

A "NO" checkmark indicates one or more of the above procedures was not accomplished safely and/or in a timely manner. You should write a very brief description of the problem and the action(s) taken to correct the deficiency. It is recommended that you re-accomplish the portion(s) or the exercise that was unsatisfactory to ensure the revised procedure(s) will work. A suggested "Tornado/ Severe Weather Procedures Exercise Record" sheet follows.

Tornado/Severe Weather Exercise Record

Blank Forms are available online. Please see Table of Contents for instructions.

Flood

Flooding is the most common natural hazard in the United States, affecting more than 20,000 local jurisdictions and representing more than 70 percent of Presidential disaster declarations. Several evaluations have estimated that seven to 10 percent of the nation's land area is subject to flooding. Some communities have very little flood risk; others lie entirely within a floodplain, or in proximity to rivers or canals.

Flooding is a natural process that may occur in a variety of forms: long-duration flooding along rivers that drain large watersheds; flash floods that send a devastating wall of water down a mountain canyon; and coastal flooding that accompanies high tides and onshore winds, hurricanes, and nor'easters. When this natural process does not affect human activity, flooding is not a problem. In fact, many species of plants and animals that live adjacent to bodies of water are adapted to a regimen of periodic flooding.

Flooding is only considered a problem when human development is located in areas prone to flooding. Such development exposes people to potentially life-threatening situations and makes property vulnerable to serious damage or destruction. It also can disrupt the natural surface flow, redirecting water onto lands not normally subject to flooding.

Flooding along waterways normally occurs as a result of excessive rainfall or snowmelt that exceeds the capacity of channels. Flooding along shorelines is usually a result of coastal storms that generate storm surges or waves above normal tidal fluctuations. Factors that can affect the frequency and severity of flooding and the resulting damage include:

▸ Channel obstructions caused by fallen trees, accumulated debris or ice jams

▸ Channel obstructions caused by road and rail crossings where the bridge or culvert openings are insufficient to convey floodwaters

▸ Erosion of shorelines and stream banks, often with episodic collapse of large areas of land

▸ Deposition of sediment that settles out of floodwaters or is carried inland by wave action

▸ Increased upland development of impervious surfaces and manmade drainage improvements that increase runoff volumes

▸ Land subsidence, which increases flood depths

▸ Failure of dams (resulting from seismic activity, lack of maintenance, flows that exceed the design or destructive acts), which may suddenly and unexpectedly release large volumes of water

▸ Failure of levees (associated with flows that exceed the design, weakening by seismic activity, lack of maintenance or destructive acts), which may result in sudden flooding of areas behind levees

▸ Failure of seawalls, revetments, bulkheads, or similar coastal structures, which can lead to rapid erosion and increased flooding and wave damage during storms

Each type of flooding has characteristics that represent important aspects of the hazard. These characteristics should be considered in the selection of hospital sites, the design of new facilities, and the expansion or rehabilitation of existing flood-prone facilities. Existing flood-prone hospitals are susceptible to damage, the nature and severity of which is a function of site-specific flood characteristics. Damage may include: site damage, structural and nonstructural building damage, destruction or impairment of utility service equipment, and loss of contents. It is important to place emergency generators above the flood zone.

 Remember ⸺⸺⸺⸺⸺

Flooding is the major cause of loss of life in hurricanes.

Regardless of the nature and severity of damage, flooded hospitals typically are not functional while cleanup and repairs are undertaken. The length of closure, and thus the impact on the ability of the facility to become operational, depends on the severity of the damage and lingering health hazards. Sometimes repairs are put on hold pending a decision on whether a hospital should be rebuilt at the flood-prone site. When damage is substantial, rehabilitation or reconstruction is allowed only if compliance with flood-resistant design requirements is achieved.

Floods can cause significant damage to facility sites, structures and utilities. Fast-flowing water causes erosion and scouring, deposits sediment and debris, destroys landscaping and fences, and can close and even wash away access roads. Other effects can be structural damage to load-bearing parts of a building while standing water can lead to damage to floors, walls and sub-structures. Even minor flooding can render a building unusable and lead to problems with mold and other forms of contamination.

Large medical equipment that is permanently installed usually is considered to be part of the building rather than contents. The nature and sensitivity of most medical equipment suggests that post-flood cleaning to restore functionality may not be feasible. This limits options for existing hospitals that use such equipment in areas that will be exposed to flooding, because temporary relocation of the equipment cannot be part of an emergency response plan.

Flood Plain Status: Select the appropriate statement shown next. If you are unsure about being in or out of a flood plain, ask your Local Emergency Management Office. This statement should be included with the CEMP for a facility. Sea, Lake and Overland Surges from Hurricanes (SLOSH) models are available as a resource to identify flood plain status.

‣   "Insert the Name of Facility" is not located in a flood plain.

‣   "Insert the Name of Facility" is located in a flood plain.

Flood Watch: Flooding is possible.

‣   Monitor National Oceanographic and Atmospheric Administration (NOAA) radio or commercial radio or TV for additional information.

‣   Be prepared to evacuate to higher ground.

Flood Warning: Flooding is occurring in your area or will occur soon.

‣   Prepare to evacuate your facility.

‣   Monitor National Oceanographic and Atmospheric Administration (NOAA) radio or commercial radio or TV.

‣   If you are paired with a facility outside the projected flood waters, you may want to evacuate before being asked to evacuate by the authorities.

‣   If you decide to evacuate your facility and go to higher ground, call and coordinate your evacuation with the Local Emergency Management Office. The roads you want to travel may already be underwater. (The Local Emergency Management Director will provide you with the number to call.)

Flash Flood Watch: Flash flooding is possible. A flash flood can occur without warning.

If your facility is in an area that has a history of flash flooding, it is strongly suggested that you use this part of the Annex to list those minimum things your staff should do when a flash flood watch is issued.

Flash Flood Warning: A flash flood is occurring.

Evacuation:

‣   Notify the administrator.

‣   Call the Local Emergency Management Agency at _____ and let them know you are evacuating your facility. (The Local Emergency Management Office will provide you with the number to call.)

‣ Ensure residents/patients carry prescription medications with them.

‣ The administrator will ensure families of employees and residents/patients are notified as necessary.

After The Flood:

‣ Do not turn on or plug in any electrical appliances until told to do so by a qualified electrician.

‣ Do not turn on gas appliances until told to do so by a qualified gas system technician.

‣ Prepare an inventory of losses associated with flooding of the facility.

‣ Take photographs and/or video footage of the facility.

‣ Report any damages and approximate dollar value to your Local Emergency Management Agency.

Exercises: This annex will be exercised at least once per calendar year. Documentation of the annual exercise will include:

‣ Date of the exercise: FLOODING exercise must be accomplished prior to MARCH each year.

‣ List the type of flooding exercise (FLOOD or FLASH FLOOD).

‣ Results of the exercise: Satisfactory: YES _____ NO _____ (Satisfactory indicates that each Procedure listed above was accomplished safely and in a timely manner.)

A "NO" check mark indicates one or more of the above procedures was not accomplished safely and/or in a timely manner. You should write a very brief description of the problem and the action(s) taken to correct the deficiency. It is recommended that you re-accomplish the portion(s) or the exercise that was unsatisfactory to ensure the revised procedure(s) will work. A suggested "Flooding Procedures Exercise Record" sheet follows.

Flooding Exercise Record

Blank Forms are available online. Please see Table of Contents for instructions.

Earthquake and Tsunami

Moderate earthquakes occur more frequently than major earthquakes. Nonetheless, moderate earthquakes can cause serious damage to building contents and nonstructural building systems, serious injury to occupants and staff, and disruption of building operations. Major earthquakes can cause catastrophic damage including structural collapse and massive loss of life. Those responsible for hospital safety must understand and manage these risks, particularly risks that threaten the lives of patients, doctors, nurses and staff.

Earthquake risk is the product of hazard exposure and building vulnerability, as shown in the following equation: RISK = HAZARD x VULNERABILITY. To manage earthquake risk in existing hospital buildings, one must understand the earthquake hazard and reduce building vulnerability. Failure to address earthquake risk leaves the health care organization exposed to potential losses, disruption, and liability for deaths and injuries. While purchasing insurance may protect the organization from financial losses and liability, it still leaves it susceptible to disruption, as well as deaths and injuries. Only building rehabilitation can reduce losses, deaths and injuries, as well as control liability and disruption; however, single-stage seismic rehabilitation can be expensive and disruptive. Incremental seismic rehabilitation can reduce that cost and disruption.

Considering Incremental Seismic Rehabilitation

The incremental rehabilitation approach to seismic risk mitigation focuses on improvements that will decrease the vulnerability of hospital buildings to earthquakes at the most appropriate and convenient times in the lifecycle of those buildings. The approach clarifies, as specifically as possible, what is the most affordable, least disruptive and most effective way to reduce seismic risk in your buildings. Prior to initiating a program of incremental seismic rehabilitation, a health care organization must first address the following three questions:

☐ Are hospital buildings located in a seismic zone?

☐ Are these buildings vulnerable to earthquakes?

☐ What can be done to reduce earthquake risk in existing vulnerable buildings?

It is possible to estimate roughly the vulnerability of a health care organization's portfolio of buildings and to identify problem buildings with a technique called "rapid visual screening." Health care organizations can produce generalized estimates of expected damage in the initial seismic risk assessment of its buildings.

Engineers have defined levels of the damage that can be expected in particular types of buildings due to varying intensities of earthquake motion. These levels of damage range from minor damage, such as cracks in walls, to total building collapse. In addition to building type, expected damage is also a function of building age and the state of maintenance. Hospitals suffering from deferred maintenance will experience greater damage than well-maintained hospitals. For example, failure to maintain masonry parapets significantly increases the possibility of life-threatening failure in even a moderate earthquake.

After initial rapid screening, specific seismic risk assessment for individual hospital buildings requires detailed engineering analysis.

Other Earthquake Losses

While a serious concern in its own right, building failure is the direct cause of even more important earthquake losses:

- Death and injury of patients, doctors, nurses, and staff
- Destruction of hospital contents and equipment
- Disruption of the delivery of all patient care services, including the capability to provide emergency services in a disaster

The expected extent of these losses can also be estimated based on hazard and vulnerability assessments.

The most important consideration for earthquake safety in hospital buildings is to reduce the risk of catastrophic structural collapse. Most likely in existing vulnerable buildings, structural collapse poses the greatest threat to life in a major earthquake. Choosing the method of protection from structural collapse in a deficient building requires two critical decisions:

Replace or Rehabilitate: If you decide to replace a building, new construction is carried out according to modern codes and can be assumed to meet current safety standards. However, financial constraints, historic preservation concerns and other community interests may make the replacement option infeasible. In that case, rehabilitation should be considered.

Single-Stage Rehabilitation or Incremental Rehabilitation: If the rehabilitation option is chosen, there are still issues of cost and disruption associated with the rehabilitation work. The cost of single-stage seismic rehabilitation has proved to be a serious impediment to its implementation by many health care organizations. Incremental seismic rehabilitation is specifically designed to address and reduce the problems of cost and disruption.

Response

> Remember: You will have no warning before an earthquake occurs.

During The Earthquake:

▸ When the shaking begins, get under the nearest piece of heavy furniture, wedge yourself in a doorway, get under a bed or in a bathtub, and hold on.

▸ Do not attempt to go outside until the shaking has stopped.

▸ Most earthquake-related injuries occur from falling objects.

▸ It is not recommended to attempt to take any action (job assignments) while an earthquake is occurring except TAKE COVER and hang on.

After The Shaking Stops:

▸ Check yourself and those near you for injuries.

▸ Perform simple rescues such as removing victims from under lightweight debris.

▸ To the best of your ability, assess the number and types of injuries at your facility.

▸ If the facility appears to be structurally unsafe, evacuate to an open outside area that is free of trees, overhead power lines, adjacent tall structures, etc. An aftershock can occur at any time and cause previously damaged buildings to collapse.

▸ Telephones may or may not work. If phones are working, do not use them unless there is a medical, fire or Hazardous Materials emergency. Using your phone may cause the system to fail.

▸ Turn off all utilities and leave them off until you are told it is safe to turn them on.

▸ All off-duty personnel should automatically report for duty if they can reach the facility safely. They should ensure their family members are safe before reporting. Do not use the phone to call in off-duty personnel.

▸ Consider post-event teleworking for non-medical staff members who cannot get to the facility.

Exercises: This annex will be exercised at least once per calendar year. Documentation of the annual exercise will include:

▸ **Date of the exercise:** (Must be exercise once per year, any time.)

▸ **List the type of exercise:** EARTHQUAKE

▸ **Results of the exercise:** Satisfactory: YES _____ NO _____ (Satisfactory indicates that each procedure listed was accomplished safely and in a timely manner.)

A "NO" check mark indicates one or more of the procedures was not accomplished safely and/or in a timely manner. You should write a very brief description of the problem and the action(s) taken to correct the deficiency. It is recommended that you re-accomplish the portion(s) or the exercise that was unsatisfactory to ensure the revised procedure(s) will work. A suggested "Earthquake Procedures Exercise Record" sheet follows.

Earthquake Exercise Record

Blank Forms are available online. Please see Table of Contents for instructions.

Biological, Chemical, Radiological (BCR)

Remember impacting events can take place both with the hospital and externally. As soon as a disaster involving a BCR event is verified, the Emergency Management Plan and the following components should be implemented. Because of radiology equipment at hospitals, the radiation safety officers play an important role.

Notification of Key Personnel

In hospitals, the activation of the HICS team and needed medical/technical specialists should occur as part of a mass notification.

In nursing homes, if the incident occurs after normal work hours, holidays or weekends, then the operator shall immediately contact these individuals at home or by pager.

A Patient Decontamination Area will be established prior to the arrival of contaminated casualties. No victim should be admitted or transported into the building without decontamination process unless the Emergency Management Group has determined that the victim presents no health or safety hazard to the facility.

Rapid Identification or Verification of the Suspected Chemical Agents

At the time of initial communication, the Emergency Department Charge Nurse will obtain information as to the type of chemical agent. Many hospitals use a team approach and have someone assigned as part of research using NIOSH, material safety data sheet, orange DOT book (ERG) and poison control, if necessary. This will be conveyed to the Incident Commander.

There may be cases where the agents are unknown or agent confirmation is warranted. If identification of the agent is not immediate or readily apparent, then response may be initiated based upon patient symptoms, using hard copy or electronic resources (CDC, ATSDR- Agency for Toxic Substances and Disease Registry), consultation with Poison Control, MSDS (Material Safety Data Sheets), EMS/Hazmat, ESF-8, other hospitals and with medical/technical specialists that are part of the Hospital Command Center team.

Establish a Definitive Plan of Action Using Available Data and Resources for Mass Casualty Management Based on the Chemical Agent

Following agent identification, an Incident Action Plan (IAP) will be developed for response. This will be presented to and approved by the Command Center Team. This will include patient, equipment and vehicular containment (as necessary), use of personal protective equipment, disposal of hazardous materials and agent containment. Available data and references will be reviewed for this purpose.

Patient vehicles can have significant contamination levels and will most likely be beyond the capabilities of the hospital to decontaminate. In past significant chemical events, vehicles had to be buried with special precautions. For hospital vehicles (removed from the scene of the chemical release), the Command Center can seek the guidance of Hazmat re: decontamination of their vehicles.

Decontamination Area

Hospitals establish their decon teams based on the size of their hospital and proximity to threats. There needs to be a team A/B or Alpha/Bravo in place to provide relief, especially in a large or sustained event. There is no prescriptive list of who should be on the team, but there must be enough people to put the plan into operation.

Anyone whose skin or clothing has been contaminated by blister or nerve agents can contaminate rescuers by direct contact or through off-gassing vapor. In the absence of agent-specific guidance, exposed areas should be cleansed using a copious amount of plain soap and water. Potentially contaminated clothing should be removed as soon as possible by staff as off gassing can occur and further contaminate personnel. However, if the chemical event is suspected to be a terrorist event, coordinate this function with outside agencies, i.e., usually local law enforcement as first responders and then the FBI as the local field office, as they may require the collection of exposed clothing and other potential evidence for submission to FBI or Department of Defense laboratories to assist in exposure investigations.

Containment of the Chemical Agents Within the Contaminated Areas

The principles of Standard Precautions must be generally applied for the management of patient-care equipment and environmental control. Rooms and bedside equipment of patients with chemical-related diseases should be cleaned using the same procedures that are used for all patients as a component of Standard Precautions, unless the contaminating chemical and the amount of environmental contamination indicates special cleaning. This also applies to soiled linen. You have to protect the building envelope and staff. One solution is to place a sign on the walk-in entrance to the hospital requesting people who have been contaminated to stay there and use the intercom provided. Hospital personnel can then go and assess the situation.

Protection of Health Care Workers

Upon completion of decontamination, each staff member involved in decontamination removes protective clothing placing all of it in red biohazard bags.

- ▸ Remove outer protective gown, turning it inside out; avoid shaking.
- ▸ Remove outer gloves first, turning them inside out as they are pulled off.
- ▸ Remove eyewear, mask and then head cover.
- ▸ Take shower per Decontamination Standard Operating Guidelines. The Decon team leader will refresh decon team staff on SOGs prior to deployment.

Agents of chemical terrorism are generally transmitted from person to person; re-aerosolization of these agents is likely. All patients, visitors and staff must be screened before entering hospital property to ensure they are not contaminated. Contaminated persons must not be allowed on hospital property at all costs until they are properly decontaminated offsite. Only decontaminated patients will be transported on designated stretchers and wheelchairs. Transport and movement of patients must be limited to that which is essential to provide patient care and follow principles of Standard Precautions.

The laboratory should be advised of the suspected biological, chemical or radiological agent involved. All autopsies must be performed applying Standard Precautions to include the use of masks and eyewear, whenever the generation of aerosols or splatter of body fluids is anticipated.

Bioterrorism agents are separated into three categories – A, B, or C – depending on how easily they can be spread and the severity of illness or death they cause. CDC Category A agents include organisms and toxins that pose the highest risk to the public and national security because they can be easily spread or transmitted from person to person, they result in high death rates, they can cause extreme concern and social disruption and they require special action for public health preparedness, i.e., smallpox, pneumonic plague and viral hemorrhagic fever, for example.

Training

Training for health care providers should include emergency management roles, responsibilities and procedures. Staff assigned to HICS or emergency response roles should take ICS training, specifically IS-100, 200, 700 and 800. In addition, such staff members need a basic CBRNE awareness-level course. In Florida, the state's Hospital Preparedness Team published the 2011 Disaster Core Competencies for Hospital Personnel. It can be located at: www.doh.state.fl.us/demo/BPR/hospprepared.html.

Local Emergency Management staff members also provide certificate courses that are usually free of charge. Facility staff should also be familiar with the different types of hazards their facility could potentially experience and how to respond in each event. They should also be knowledgeable of the various medical conditions and mobility impairments affecting their patients and know where/how to access the patient records for use during and after emergency evacuations.

Types of Training

Following is a summary of the different types of training available to enhance staff performance during a disaster response:

American Red Cross Training

The American Red Cross (ARC) offers a variety of training materials and courses for individual, family, organization and business preparedness.

The Salvation Army

The local Salvation Army Corps Center may be contacted for information on their training and resource programs.

Local/State Emergency Management Programs

Most states have many emergency management training programs to assist the public and private sector in preparing for emergencies. Training available includes a wide variety of emergency management courses for city, county and state government administrators, as well as highly specialized courses geared for practicing law and fire professionals.

Federal Emergency Management Programs

The Federal Emergency Management Agency (FEMA) provides a variety of opportunities for continuing education as part of their Professional Training Program. Their methods of instruction include home study and classroom courses. Some are provided locally at colleges or other FEMA authorized institution. FEMA in Anniston, Alabama, has great programs, as does the National Fire Academy in Maryland.

Chemical Spills Procedures Plan

This section is designed to address a Hazardous Materials (Chemical Spill) inside your facility, outside on facility property and in the vicinity of the facility.

Reporting Hazardous Materials (Chemical) Spills: Incidents/accidents involving Hazardous Materials (substances) must be reported to the appropriate local and state authorities. This is usually accomplished through the Local Emergency Management Agency or the Fire Department. (Check with your Local Emergency Management Office to determine how reporting is managed in your county/city.

Minor Spills Inside Facility Or On Property Outside:

Use resources such as MSDS (Material Safety Data Sheets), DOT Emergency Response Guide, CDC Chem Agent List and ATSDR. Hospitals should have internal response teams for spills, trained to the HAZWOPER level:

▸ Isolate (evacuate) the immediate area, and call 911.

▸ DO NOT touch, inhale or perform taste tests on the spilled material.

▸ Provide first response units with as much information as you can about the material, spill circumstances and location.

Major Spills Inside Facility And/Or On Property Outside:

Use resources such as MSDS (Material Safety Data Sheets), DOT Emergency Response Guide, CDC Chemical Agents List and ATSDR. Hospitals should have internal response teams for spills, trained to the HAZWOPER level:

▸ Isolate (evacuate) the area, and call 911.

▸ DO NOT touch, inhale or perform taste tests on the spilled material.

▸ Provide first response units with as much information as you can about the material, spill circumstances and location.

▸ If possible, move everyone uphill and upwind.

▸ Be prepared to move (evacuate) employees and residents/patients to a paired facility or location designated by Local Emergency Management personnel.

Every health care facility is vulnerable to a Hazardous Materials incident/accident because of one or more of the following:

▸ Located within one mile of a railroad

▸ Located within one mile of a county, state or federal highway

▸ Uses propane gas from 500 gallon or larger tank

▸ Uses natural gas supplied through an underground line

▸ Regularly uses Hazardous Materials/Substances in treatment of patients

▸ Located within two (2) miles of an airport

Exercises: This annex will be exercised at least once per calendar year. Documentation of the annual exercise will include:

‣ **Date of the exercise:** (Must be exercise once per year, any time.)

‣ **List the type of exercise:** CHEMICAL SPILL

‣ **Results of the exercise:** Satisfactory: YES _____ NO _____ (Satisfactory indicates that each procedure listed was accomplished safely and in a timely manner.)

A "NO" checkmark indicates one or more of the above procedures was not accomplished safely and/ or in a timely manner. You should write a very brief description of the problem and the action(s) taken to correct the deficiency. It is recommended that you re-accomplish the portion(s) or the exercise that was unsatisfactory to ensure the revised procedure(s) will work. A suggested "Chemical Spill Procedures Exercise Record" sheet follows.

Chemical Spill Exercise Record

Blank Forms are available online. Please see Table of Contents for instructions.

Disaster Levels and Hospital Response to a Mass Casualty Incident

The Uniform Pre-Hospital Multiple Casualty Incident Procedure Predetermined Response Plan, January 2006, is considered the standard for determining disaster levels. It is available at: www.myfloridacfo.com/sfm/FOG/2006Chapter14.pdf.

The Uniformed Pre-Hospital Multiple Casualty Incident Procedure Predetermined Response Plan classifies MCIs by levels according to the actual or estimated number of casualties. The number is calculated on the initial scene "size-up" prior to EMS triage and helps to determine if additional assistance is needed from other EMS providers. It also serves as a scalable mechanism for the Incident Commander or local Communications Center to notify the closest hospitals, trauma centers and Emergency Management. According to this standard, there are five levels. The incoming number of casualties may be easily accommodated for a larger hospital, almost like an ordinary day. However, rural hospitals activate their MCI emergency code often with less than 10 patients coming in simultaneously. A higher level of acuity requires more resources.

Patient Care Units

A major component in a disaster event that requires the care of victims in a Mass Casualty Incident situation is the immediate response of the Patient Care Units and professional/licensed nursing personnel. Hospitals have electronic census reports so an assessment can be made quickly of bed availability. It might require a fast real-time update, but this can be accomplished quickly. Hospitals also have patient flow coordinators that are aware of their current bed availability and can quickly calculate this. On off-tours, the nursing supervisor is aware of bed availabilities. Also, hospitals use software programs for staffing and are aware of their staffing levels. One of the initial requests in a community disaster is a request by the local EOC for bed availabilities to be reported. This is done using HAvBED national standards. The response includes:

▸ The current available staffing to meet the incoming needs of the victims and the current patient population in the hospital

▸ The timeframe for calling additional staffing to assist the preparation of the Surgical Suites

Nursing Units are requested to follow the list of instructions and provide the appropriate information to the Command Center on notification or announcement of a disaster situation or emergency event.

All patient care staff will immediately return to their home unit.

The physicians must be involved to determine if patients can be discharged of transferred. The medical staff needs to receive a mass notification through the Medical Staff Office to conduct this review for who can be discharged, etc. Case managers are very helpful to support the arrangements. A discharge holding area can be used as a transition area while families are notified.

 Must Do ━━━━━━━

Hospitals should have electronic processes to adjust staffing.

The department director and next shift supervisor should be notified by the staff during the recall process. It is worth considering a disaster hotline and many hospitals are adopting mass notification systems for self-enrollment similar to college campuses. The most reliable method to date is a pager and text message for notice to the entire management team.

For a Level I event, do not activate the Disaster Recall List to call in additional department associates unless notified by the Command Center to do so. For a Level II or III event, the associate recall should be implemented. All associates on the Recall List should be called back to work based on availability and proximity to the hospital. All associates scheduled for the immediate next shift should be asked to come in to the hospital.

The Incident Command System should be implemented. The Planning Chief will work with the Operations Chief in the Command Center to determine what is needed for staffing based on the size or acuity levels of the disaster. They will assign a designee to call staff to come in. All incoming staff should report to the staff staging area to sign in and to be assigned where needed. Documentation of staffing signing in/out- electronically, or on paper, is critical to request reimbursement from FEMA after a disaster.

Staffing will be assessed by the Nurse Director, and the number of staff available for reassignment will be specified. When notified by the Command Center, expendable staff should be sent to the staffing pool. In Florida, a system has been set up with job descriptions for green, red, yellow and black station nurses.

Bed Control will begin calling each unit with anticipated admissions. Hospitals are now using hospitalists and intensivists that have a significant role in admitting, discharging and transferring patients.

Evaluate current supplies and equipment on-hand that would be used for day-to-day operations. Hospitals may carry up to three days' supply, with more available at the CSCA distribution center.

Triage And Trauma Center and Emergency Department

For incoming patients, triage is critical in determining treatment needed, transportation required and most suitable receiving facility.

Pre-Event Actions

Receiving information about an impending emergency event or incident could significantly impact the Emergency Department and Trauma Center. This information serves to provide an outline for patient management in the event of an internal or external disaster, since the initial and greatest impact will be on the facility's emergency services. It also provides for a process for the efficient management of patient flow and provision of safe care during a disaster event or emergency situation. Examples of such events could be the volume of patients exceeding the physical space and resources, or the arrival of multiple patients within a short period of time.

Charge Nurse

When the charge nurse is notified of multiple patients arriving due to an emergency event or Mass Casualty Incident, the actions taken will be as follows:

▸ Notify the Administrator on call first. HICS activation will be determined to the level needed. Sometimes it is just the Incident Commander or the Command Center team that is required to support an incident. HICS is intended to be flexible and adaptable to the incident and scalable to the level that is needed. Hospitals include the ED Director and Safety Officers in their direct notifications.

What does your plan say? A good strategy is for mass notification of all management team members.

Inform all Emergency Department (ED) and Trauma Services staff and physicians and Lead Registration of the situation/scenario and tentative plan of action. Evaluate staffing in all ED and

Trauma areas and determine if more staff needs to be called in. Discuss with ED and Trauma Physician(s) working if the coverage is sufficient to meet the volume of patients, and determine if the on-call physician needs to be called.

Initial Assessment and Triage

Triage is a process of sorting out casualties to assess their acuity level and priority for care. An assessment method is used to facilitate this (START and JumpSTART). Casualties can arrive at an ED without having been triaged (so they will need an initial assessment). EMS transported casualties should receive a reassessment by ED personnel to update their status.

▸ Upon assessment and labeling of victims of a disaster situation or emergency event at the scene or in the pre-hospital environment, the initial assessment of the victim continues on arrival to the essential patient care areas.

▸ Upon arrival to the hospitals, an initial TRIAGE occurs by the Triage Officer to:

▷ Identify incoming patients by color of the bracelet or triage tag assessment.

▷ Establish treatment priorities based on the color of the bracelet or triage tag assessment.

▷ Assign the patient to the appropriate patient care area. Green tagged – minor care – casualties can be assigned to a clinic or Alternate Care Site.

▷ Begin the registration process.

Preparation of Triage Area

The function of the triage sites include assessing all sick and injured, sending them to the appropriate essential patient care areas as designated in the Patient Care Locations, and assisting in transporting the victims appropriately.

Transport all stretchers and wheelchairs from within the department, gather additional as needed from Clinical Transport associates, and assemble essential extra supplies in Triage Area from Central Supply. Then send to internal or external areas as needed to address surge – if warranted.

Cape Canaveral Hospital received notification that it would receive had 500 patients from one cruise ship event while in another – although initial reports warned it would be hosting 1,800 patients – only 120 sought treatment.

Patient Representative

Inform the patients and families that the ED is going to be receiving victims from a disaster or emergency event. Consequently, there may be delays in receiving medical care.

Inform the social worker on call of the anticipated patient volume into the ED and support that is anticipated to be needed.

Consider pastoral care and a victims' network.

Registration

Casualties of a disaster situation or emergency event (as already stated) can be tagged in the pre-hospital environment with a bracelet – red, yellow, green or black (they may also be tagged in the pre-hospital environment or at the ED of a hospital or an ACS). All walk-ins will receive triage but not necessarily a triage tag.

Most hospitals have pre-identified medical record numbers that can be used for disaster casualties. When the casualty arrives at the triage sites, the registration associates use this number as part of the numerical identification of the patient by "Hospital Number." The triage tag number should be listed on the Master Log of Disaster Casualties, and the Medical Record Number is also listed (as well as in the patient's chart); hospitals are now using EMRs (Electronic Medical Records,) and the future will be that the patient's triage tag with a barcoded triage tag number will be scanned as part of patient tracking into a log and can also be inserted in the chart to link it with the medical record. Some ED tracking boards can identify the incident (Train Crash, Bus Crash, Tornado, etc.); however, when there are multiple simultaneous events, as in a catastrophic level disaster, it is important not to lump them all together. While the ED tracking board can do this (if someone inputs each of the various events), the "Hospital Number"/Medical Record Number may not be able to reflect all of this info.

Some hospitals have Disaster Census Screens; this would be a best practice example, but not all hospitals may have this capability.

The hospital medical record number is the one used for billing.

Staffing

Emergency Department nurses and an Emergency Department Physician will staff the triage area as deemed necessary by the Treatment Area Supervisor (TAS) although small hospitals may not have a TAS. You need to staff both the ambulatory entry area (bolstering triage staff there) and the ambulance entrance.

Triage staff members typically include an RN and an ED technician. In large academic medical centers, they may also staff triage with a physician (attending or resident, possibly). In smaller hospitals, the ED physician is needed to care for patients (and to complete dispositions of those who can be discharged or will be admitted) to clear bed availability.

Emergency Department Management Actions

▸ The ED Management or designee will ensure the following actions are completed:

▹ Designate and staff the ambulatory and ambulance entry area with Triage staff including at a minimum ED RN, ED technician and Registration Associate. Ambulatory self-transported casualties may arrive well before EMS transported ones. You need to staff both the ambulatory (bolstering staff there) and the ambulance entry area. Request ED physician to work with triage nurse at ambulance entrance to assess red-tagged casualties in need of immediate care.

▷ Consider tele-triage. This has been done successfully on a number of occasions and is a goal of the State of Florida trauma network. This has saved countless lives on the battlefields of Iraq and Afghanistan.

▷ Request the ED physician to work with a second Triage Nurse to evaluate the patient's condition.

▷ Bring a Triage Supply Cart to the ambulance Triage Area. This should contain vital signs assessment equipment, hemorrhagic control supplies and PPE for staff. Also hospitals might need to staff and supply a 3rd Triage Area for non-disaster ambulatory casualties. Supply carts are usually labeled green, yellow and red to correspond with Start to Finish locations on your campus.

▷ Bring the MCI supply cart to the ED triage staging area. It should be stocked with initial critical items (vests, first aid supplies, disaster charts, cones, caution tape, bullhorn, flashlights), rapid response kits (large color-coded tarps matching disaster colors – often with matching flags, vest and manifest clipboards) and other supplies – litters, extra lighting, respiratory supplies, etc. You could also consider creating an electronic version of appropriate items.

▷ Designate staff as communication support to answer internal and external phones, radios, beepers, etc. Note: Communications support staff members are needed in the hospital Operators area, ED, Command Center and Family Assistance Area. Having support in the ED is important, as multiple communication devices all go off at once; the Charge Nurse has the responsibility for communicating info to the AOC (administrator on call), or to the Command Center, and is tied up with that.

▷ Designate someone to call in additional staff and/or physicians if needed.

Prehospital S.T.A.R.T.

▸ **S.T.A.R.T. (Simple Triage and Rapid Transport).** Pre-hospital providers are taught how to assess Airway-Breathing-Circulation (ABCs) in patients, which makes teaching them to use the model easier and translates to a rapid assessment method. There are several advantages to using the S.T.A.R.T.

▷ It is simple to learn and use in the field. Most of all, pre-hospital providers are taught how to perform the ABCs of patient care. The S.T.A.R.T. Plan follows the ABCs, thereby making it rapid to perform.

▷ It allows for immediate stabilization of life-threatening airway and bleeding problems.

▸ The S.T.A.R.T. Plan uses three (3) criteria to categorize victims:

▷ Ventilation

▷ Perfusion

▷ Mental Status

▸ **1:** The initial medical responder enters the incident area, identifies him/herself and directs all the victims who can walk to gather and remain at an identified point. This identifies those victims who presently have sufficient respiratory, circulatory and neuro-motor functions enough to walk. Most of these victims will be triaged green; however, they are not tagged at this time, but triaged separately later.

▸ **2:** Begin evaluation of the first non-ambulatory victims where they are lying. Assess the victim's ventilation. Is it normal, rapid, or absent? If respiration is absent, reposition the airway to see if breathing begins. If respiration remains absent, tag black. Do not perform CPR. If the victim requires help in maintaining an open airway or has a respiration rate over 30 per minute, tag red. (Attempt to utilize non-EMS person to hold the airway). If respirations are normal (less than 30 per minute), go to the next step.

▸ **3:** Assess victim's perfusion. Perfusion can be assessed by performing the capillary refill test or by palpating a radial pulse. If the capillary refill is over two seconds or if the radial pulse is absent, tag red. If the capillary refill is less than two seconds, or if the radial pulse is present, go on to the next step. Any life-threatening bleeding should be controlled immediately. Elevate the victim's legs to begin shock treatment. (Again, attempt to utilize a non-EMS person to maintain pressure at the bleeding site).

During The Event

Bed Requests

▸ Bed request assignments are generally done through an electronic process in hospitals. When a notification occurs that there is an event, assigning beds for admitted patients in the ED is a priority. Using the HICS structure, the Operations Chief should be aware of the need to free up beds in the ED by assigning beds for those who are already admitted or anticipated to need admission. There needs to be communication with the ED Charge Nurse to expedite the process. The electronic patient tracking boards and pager systems for bed requests will detail the kind of beds that are needed.

Triage

▸ Initial assessment of patients will be performed by the triage staff. An Emergency Department Treatment Record will be initiated with Identification data and "Chief Complaint."

▸ Triage of ambulatory victims and others that arrive by private vehicle will be done at the main walk-in entrance to the Emergency Department by a Triage Team as already stated. Registration associates will also be assigned to this area. Triage of ambulance and seriously ill patients brought by other vehicles will be performed in the Ambulance Entrance.

▸ Patients will be transported to and managed in the essential patient care areas. The Treatment Area Supervisor may reassign or re-prioritize patients at any time based on changes in condition or the current or anticipated needs of the victims.

▸ The Treatment Area Supervisor or alternate management designee will coordinate the placement of all patients after they are triaged. There should be one Master Log for an event that gets updated as frequently as possible. Primary Triage will more likely keep one half of the perforated triage tag that designates the acuity level of each patient. As patients get registered, a label from their patient medical record can be affixed to the Master Log. This way, each patients name, gender and DOB will all be displayed on each label. The Treatment Area Supervisor will obtain a copy of this every 30 minutes, so as to have an accurate list of victims. The list of victims will be delivered to the Command Center every hour or sooner, if requested.

▸ The Treatment Area Supervisor, Management and ED Physician will, each hour, review the status of all ED patients to determine who can be discharged, admitted or moved to another ED location. The Charge Nurse and ED physician will review patients in the ED treatment area and waiting room. The following will be determined:

   ▷ Which patients need to be admitted quickly?

   ▷ Which patients need to be discharged?

   ▷ Which patients need to be moved to another section of the ED; this will include the patients that can be moved to the waiting room?

   ▷ What needs to happen with the patients in the waiting room?

The triage nurse in the ambulatory entry area will direct the ED Technician to obtain repeat vital signs as a reassessment for each patient in the waiting room during the Disaster Event. This information and any changes in patient condition will need to be communicated to the Primary Triage Nurse who will then inform the Treatment Area Supervisor if a patient's condition in the waiting room has changed and warrants being brought back to the treatment area.

Emergency Department Management

The Management person or designee will be the primary communicator and is responsible to up date all ED staff and physicians regarding the event and the plan. The Command Center Liaison Officer will function as a liaison between the ED Charge Nurse, the ED and the Hospital Command Center.

Operations

The Treatment Area Supervisor will communicate any needs for additional support to the Command Center Liaison Officer and will continually re-evaluate the department's status for staffing, supplies, etc., in order to deliver safe and efficient care during the event.

Post-Event

Emergency Department Management

The Treatment Area Supervisor or designee will inform all of the ED staff and physicians that the casualties have all been received. Collaboratively, the Administrative and Medical Directors or designees will determine when the ED will return to normal patient flow operations and communicate this to all staff and physicians. This information also needs to be communicated to the support services within the department, i.e., Registration, Radiology, etc. Additionally this information needs to be communicated to the Command Center Liaison Officer.

Operation

ED assignments and patient flow will be transitioned back to normal operations. Staffing will be evaluated and additional staff will be released, as appropriate.

Emergency Department Volume Overload

Receiving information about an impending emergency event or incident could significantly impact the Emergency Department and Trauma Center. It's also possible for the Emergency Department to be stressed due to a surge in patients as part of a seasonal surge, or for unexplained reasons as part of a higher-volume day. This type of situation must be addressed, but is not normally considered a disaster or MCI type of situation. The following information serves to provide an outline for patient management in the event of an unexpected surge in Emergency Department patient levels. It quantifies "Trigger" levels to implement a process for the efficient management of patient flow and provision of safe care during the event.

The following describes the procedure at one large regional medical center:

Trigger #1

Will be implemented when the bed availability criteria reaches the following limit (Combination of any 3)

ICU:	3 beds
PCU:	5 beds
Med/Surg:	5 beds
ED Holds:	5 Pts>2 Hrs
PACU Holds:	5 Pts>5 Hrs

The following actions will be taken for Trigger #1: (an example from one hospital)

▸ Patient Care Services will identify "Adopt a Boarder" patients.

▸ Bed Control will initiate stand-by list of Direct Admits.

▸ Case Management and First Flight will not accept most transfers from non-Health First facilities.

▸ Case Management, Bed Control and Patient Care Services will open and use the Discharge Holding Area.

▸ Bed Control and Patient Care Services will ensure an assessment of potential ED Admits.

▸ Case Management, Bed Control and Patient Care Services will prioritize transport and bed clean activities.

▸ Patient Care Services will ensure the Charge Nurses expedite discharges.

The following positions will be notified by pager:

▸ Bed Control Manager

▸ Administrator On Call

▸ Nurse Managers and Clinical Charge Nurses and Directors

▸ Ancillary Department Managers

▸ Staffing Office calls On-Call staff for potential opening of the Overflow Units.

Trigger #2

Will be implemented when the bed availability criteria reaches the following limit (Combination of any 3).

ICU: 2 beds

PCU: 3 beds

Med/Surg: 3 beds

ED Holds: 8 Pts>2 Hrs

PACU Holds: 5 Pts>2 Hrs

The following actions will be taken for Trigger #2:

▸ Outpatient surgery center patients requiring admission are placed in PACU holding.

▸ Patient Care Services will assess Overflow Unit capabilities (GI, Lab, PICU, PACU, Flex, Rad Holding and Cath Staging).

▸ Case Management will alert Ancillary Dept and Central Services to assess staffing and service level needs, i.e., Rad/Lab/PT.

▸ Case Management and Patient Care Services will place calls to physicians to schedule non-emergent studies to facilitate early discharge.

The following positions will be notified by pager:

▸ Medical Staff Officers

▸ Nursing Directors

▸ CNO

▸ AOC

▸ Vice President Safety and Security

▸ Vice President Medical Affairs

▸ UR Director

▸ Case Management Director

Trigger #3

Will be implemented when the bed availability criteria reaches the following limit (Combination of any 3).

ICU:	1 bed
PCU:	2 beds
Med/Surg:	2 beds
ED Holds:	10 Pts>2 Hrs
PACU Holds:	10 Pts>2 Hrs

The following actions will be taken for Trigger #3:

‣ AOC, Patient Care Services and Bed Control implement "adopt a boarder."

‣ Case Management and Patient Care Services activate additional staffing and open overflow units.

‣ Case Management, UR Director and Surgery activate stand-by list for direct admits and initiate triage list for elective surgeries.

‣ Emergency Department will consider diversion.

‣ Case Management and UR Director will activate ancillary departments to increase staffing service levels, i.e., Rad/Lab/PT.

‣ COO will ensure all Matrix Managers are onsite.

‣ Patient Care Services will mobilize non-clinical nursing staff.

‣ Patient Care Services will close the GI Lab and cancel elective GIs. Consider using this area for overflow.

The following positions will be notified by pager:

‣ Medical Staff Officers

‣ Nursing, Case Management and non-clinical Directors

‣ CNO, COO, CEO, VPSS/VPMA/UR Director

‣ Community physicians by group fax from the Med Staff Office

‣ Notify PBCH and CCH of situation

‣ Matrix Managers

‣ Ancillary Directors

‣ Human Resources

‣ Directors Patient Relation

‣ VP Customer Service

Trigger #4

Will be implemented when the bed availability criteria reaches the following limit (Combination of any 3).

ICU:	0 beds
PCU:	0 beds
Med/Surg:	0 beds
ED Holds:	15 Pts>2 Hrs
PACU Holds:	15 Pts>2 Hrs

The following actions will be taken for Trigger #4:

▸ AOC, Case Management, Bed Control and First Flight will ensure that the hospital is closed to admissions and transfers from other non-Health First facilities.

▸ Emergency Department will remain on diversion until off of Trigger #4.

▸ Case Management and UR Director will oversee stabilization and transfer of patients to other facilities.

▸ Case Management, AOC and Surgery will evaluate canceling elective surgeries.

▸ Human Resources will mobilize non-clinical nursing staff.

▸ Human Resources will evaluate mandatory nursing call-in.

▸ AOC will set up a modified HEICS in the Bed Control area.

The following positions will be notified by pager:

▸ Medical Staff Officers

▸ Nursing Directors

▸ CNO, COO, CEO

▸ VPSS/VPMA/UR Director

▸ Marketing Director

▸ Community physicians by group fax from the Med Staff Office

Developing a Plan, Procedures, Training and Testing

To ensure that decisions about evacuation will be completed in a timely manner, a series of inter-related actions must be addressed.

First, with input from local emergency services authority, facility planners should develop a succinct plan that describes their organization's evacuation policy, with basic information about who is in charge during evacuation, what the known risks and hazards are, and the expectations of staff and clients during and after evacuation. The plan should include agreements made with other facilities for evacuation support.

Second, a specific checklist of actions should be developed into a brief, clearly written procedure for making decisions about evacuation and implementing those decisions.

Third, staff must be trained around the plan and procedures, including a walk-through of the facility and its evacuation-related sites and equipment. This should be part of a new employee's orientation training.

Finally, the staff should be involved in, at a minimum, a tabletop evacuation exercise each year as part of the facility's licensure requirements. See NFPA requirements under emergency management, as well as The Joint Commission (TJC) and DNV. There should be hard copies, as well as online versions. Updates should be made to the online version.

Developing a Maintenance Process

Facility management should include an annex to the evacuation plan dealing with the maintenance of evacuation readiness. This should include plan and procedure revisions, training qualifications, facility readiness checklists, phone number verifications, and supplies and equipment inventory/replacement.

Health First hospitals have a poster in the command center with all the back door numbers of hospitals, local DOH, EOC and so on. It is updated each year prior to hurricane season which starts on June 1.

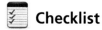 **Checklist**

Suggested Supply List

Supplies are now unit-dosed. Anticipate dosages for newborn to geriatric ages. Categories of supplies should be grouped to ensure that everything needed is included. For example: Wound Care Supplies; Medications; Diabetic Supplies; Respiratory Supplies; Pediatric Supplies, etc.

For example:

☐ Acetominophen ☐ Anaphylactic Kit ☐ Antacids ☐ Antibiotic Ointment unit-dose packets ☐ Antihistamines ☐ Aspirin 81 mg ☐ Betadine ☐ Hydrocortisone 2.5% ointment ☐ Hydrogen peroxide ☐ Insulin pens/syringes ☐ Ipecac ☐ Petrolatum ☐ KY Jelly- unit dose packets	☐ Identification bracelets; ☐ Irrigation Kit: 10 (in case there are persons with nasogastric or PEG tubes); ☐ Loop masks ☐ Magic markers; ☐ Obstetrical kit; ☐ Oxygen tanks and oxygen delivery supplies: cannulas, masks, nebulizer equipment
☐ Pediatric supplies to include: bottles, nipples, formulas, water, diapers - assorted sizes, baby wipes, Soybean formula; ☐ Bandages: assortment; ☐ Bariatric supplies; ☐ Betadine scrub lotion; ☐ Bio-hazard waste bags; ☐ Blankets; ☐ Body lotion; ☐ Bug repellant;	☐ Petroleum: unit dose packets versus a tube; ☐ Paper cups and plates; ☐ Pillows; ☐ Portable oximeter; ☐ Safety pins; ☐ Scissors; ☐ Sharps containers; ☐ Soap;
☐ Calamine lotion: suggest not including; ☐ Chlorine bleach; ☐ Colostomy bags; ☐ Commodes; ☐ Cots: regular and adjustable; ☐ Cotton balls; ☐ Diabetic supplies: Blood glucose strips, glucometer; ☐ Eye pads: eye wash; ☐ Flashlight and batteries; ☐ Forceps; ☐ Gloves: sterile;	☐ Sphygmomanometer: large adult, adult, small adult and child sizes; ☐ Splints; ☐ Sterile water; ☐ Stethoscope; ☐ Surface wipes; ☐ Thermometers: 10 and also need thermometer disposable covers (at least 100); ☐ Tongue depressors; ☐ Tourniquet; ☐ Urinary drainage catheters and bag; ☐ Wound care supplies: steristrips and Bandaids, 2x2 and 4x4 gauze pads; Adhesive tape, recommend 1" and 3" silk and paper tape; Antiseptic, Chlorhexidine unit-dose packets.

Off-campus Locations

It is important to plan in advance for off-campus locations in the event of an evacuation or major casualty incident. Off-campus locations can be a neighboring hospital, local school or any facility where health and medical services can be provided.

Setting up a Health and Medical Annex

In an emergency it may be necessary to set up temporary health and medical facilities. As part of your emergency planning you should investigate suitable sites in advance and have protocols, procedures and equipment in place in order to be able to respond rapidly whenever necessary.

Health and medical services include: emergency medical (EMS), hospital, public health, environmental health, mental-health services and mortuary services. The activities associated with these services include treatment, transport and evacuation of the injured; disposition of the dead; and disease control activities related to sanitation, preventing contamination of water and food supplies, etc., during response operations and in the aftermath of a disaster. Depending on needs and resources, jurisdictions may want to prepare separate annexes for one or more of these health and medical services.

Points to bear in mind:

- The annex applies primarily to large-scale emergency and disaster events that would cause sufficient casualties and/or fatalities to overwhelm local medical, health and mortuary services capabilities, thus requiring maximum coordination and efficient use of these resources.

- Public and private medical, health and mortuary services resources located in the jurisdiction will be available for use during disaster situations.

- Large-scale emergencies and disaster threat situations (earthquakes, hurricanes, nuclear power plant accidents, floods, etc.) may affect large areas of the jurisdiction of one or several states, requiring the use of mutual aid.

- Public and private health and medical resources located in the jurisdiction generally will be available for use during disaster situations, but many of these resources, including human resources, will themselves be impacted by the disaster.

- Emergency measures to protect life and health during the first 12 to 24 hours after the disaster in all likelihood will be exclusively dependent upon local and area resources.

- Resources available through area and regional medical, health and mortuary services mutual aid agreements will be provided for use during the disaster situation.

- It may be necessary to relocate hospital facilities under austere conditions to contingency field hospitals, or to permanent or temporary buildings that will provide patients and medical staff adequate protection from the effects of the disaster.

- Volunteers will come forward to help perform essential tasks; their efforts must be anticipated and coordinated.

www.GTIBookstore.com

Nursing Homes

In the recent past, the elderly and persons with disabilities have often been the most negatively affected by the consequences of a major disaster. The U.S. Centers for Disease Control determined that the elderly accounted for only 15 percent of New Orleans' 2005 population, but 70 percent of the deaths from Hurricane Katrina. In addition, at least 139 storm-related fatalities were reported from nursing homes as a result of Katrina. The disastrous storms of 2004-05 highlighted the consequences of the planning failure to integrate nursing homes into a national disaster response system.

A summit convened by the Florida Health Care Association of national and state leaders from long-term care, emergency management, transportation, energy, medicine and state and federal regulatory agencies, made the following recommendations.

- Nursing home disaster plans should be uniformly organized with common elements and terminology. All too often, the organization and content of disaster plans vary greatly from facility to facility, making them difficult to review and critique, and sometimes difficult to execute.

- Make sure your regulatory agency understands your plans for evacuation or sheltering in place. Do not assume that a regulatory agency will approve of your plans for evacuation or sheltering in place. Present your facility's plan to the appropriate overseer in advance to be sure it is acceptable. Note that all will want to make sure that a plan exists, but due to the responsibility and liability of approving a plan, a checkmark in the "has a plan" box may be the extent of the review.

- Assess the lifetime of your supplies on hand. Accurately assess the length of time the facility's supplies will last. The clock begins to tick on the first day of contra-flow, when suppliers have stopped coming in to your community or city.

- Conduct drills using your disaster plan. Every plan must be tested, and drills create experience and first-hand knowledge about the efficacy of a plan. Test your plans in your own facility.

- Plan for the needs of special patient groups, with special concerns for persons on dialysis. Special consideration is required for managing dialysis residents. Contact the End Stage Renal Disease (ESRD) network serving your geographic area for disaster planning assistance for the needs of dialysis patients.

- Nursing home plans need to include security strategies. Security measures are needed to protect the facility and its residents and staff during a disaster when, due to emergency generator support requirements, the facility is probably one of few buildings with food, water and medical supplies. Hospitals already have security departments and are positioned to manage such dangers, but nursing homes are not.

Evacuation Decision Making

Who makes the decision to evacuate and when is a major issue. Evacuation decisions could be rendered by the facility administrator and/or owner; the local emergency operations center; a state office; or the governor. The decision could also be made jointly by the local emergency operations director and the owner of a facility. There is strong agreement that sheltering in place is the preferable decision except for facilities in a known surge zone in an anticipated path of a hurricane. However, the decisions are complicated by many factors, including resident acuity levels, the facility's location in the surge zone, its capacity to withstand hurricane force winds and the uncertainty of the landfall area. The emergency management mantra is "run from the surge; hide from the wind," but each facility must evaluate, for each disaster event, the risks associated with a decision to evacuate versus shelter in place.

▸ Determine the facility's location in the storm surge zone, and evaluate its impact. While storm surge zone flooding has been specifically discussed, other flooding risks must also be evaluated (facility's flood zone location).

▸ Determine the facility's capacity to withstand hurricane winds. Use the information to both harden the facility as a mitigation strategy and to consider as a factor in the decision to evacuate.

▸ Impact of resident acuity levels on evacuation decision making. How many residents are on ventilators? How many have dementia or Alzheimer's disease? How many are dialysis patients? How many, for reasons of frailty or end-of-life issues, should not be moved? Analyzing the resident population by acuity level should help decision makers determine the order of evacuation and perhaps allow for partial evacuations. It was suggested that those with the highest-risk factors be evacuated, e.g., those on dialysis, while those needing custodial care might shelter in place.

▸ Evaluate the receiving facility. Does the nursing home have an agreement with a receiving facility, and is it one that the regulatory agency will accept? Can an agreement with a "like facility" be secured to receive your residents if an evacuation is necessary? If not, will your residents be able to sleep on mattresses on the floor or cots? Can you send staff with your residents? These issues must all be considered when evaluating a potential receiving facility.

▸ Make sure you understand the role and capacity of special needs shelters in your community. Determine whether special needs shelters exist in your area, and, if so, are they appropriate settings for your residents. Can you evacuate residents to a special needs shelter, if staff accompany them? Is the shelter appropriate for dialysis patients or those with Alzheimer's disease?

▸ Mandatory evacuations – timing is everything. The lack of time to evacuate can result in a default decision to shelter in place. The emergency management office issuing the mandatory evacuation will notify health care facilities in advance so that they may evacuate early. Some states have requested this consideration, but advance notice has not been granted in any state.

▸ Factor in evacuation transport time. The time it will take to evacuate patients/residents and the transportation method, coupled with resident acuity levels, also factor into the evacuation decision.

▸ Shelter in place, if at all possible. There were many voices of support for sheltering in place rather than evacuation if the facility is not at risk of storm surge flooding. While there are many factors to consider, such as the availability of supplies and staff, the primary factors are the physical structure's ability to withstand hurricane winds and access to power. Being prepared to shelter in place can require a significant financial investment; some Florida owners reported having committed millions of dollars to facility hardening. Instead of an all or nothing approach, owners might consider hardening specific sections of a facility.

Interagency Relationships

▸ Health care facilities must be a part of the disaster response system. Nursing home providers will benefit greatly from an established relationship with their local EOC offices. Become an active voice for LTC at the local emergency management office, mirroring the relationship that now exists in most coastal states where there is a "seat" at the EOC for a long-term care nursing home representative.

▸ Strong interagency partnerships create synergy for improved disaster planning, response and recovery. All coastal states' nursing home associations have worked diligently to develop and strengthen relationships with their state and regulatory agencies and ESF-8 offices. Among the results of these relationship are statewide databases for tracking the status of NHs during disasters, increasing the ability of the partners (e.g., regulatory agencies and ESF-8 personnel) to identify NHs with critical needs and increasing the efficiency of resource allocation. The American Health Care Association has worked closely with the U. S. Departments of Health and Human Services, Homeland Security and Transportation for improved relationships on behalf of long-term care providers and residents.

▸ Ensure that nursing homes are considered part of the critical infrastructure for power restoration. Working through local and state ESF-8 offices, nursing home associations and their representatives serving in local EOCs are in a unique position to educate emergency managers regarding the high-risk health status of nursing home residents and to communicate critical needs of nursing homes in the disaster area.

▸ Problem identification and resolution must be approached from an interagency perspective. The value of an interdisciplinary or interagency approach to both the identification of problems and possible solutions cannot be overstated. In almost every report of achievements, success was dependent upon an interagency/interdisciplinary approach to both defining the exact nature of the problem, and its parameters and possible solutions.

▸ Invite a pharmaceutical provider to join the emergency preparedness discussion. The access to an accurate list of each resident's medications, along with the availability of the medications, is critical. One story shared was of a group of residents who arrived at a receiving facility with one large bag filled with medications, but no instructions unique to each resident.

▸ Ensure that policymakers and legislative contacts are informed about the needs of LTC residents and the results of interagency relationships in your area. Public policy and legislative solutions are more effective and successful when they are an expression of the work of informed and committed partners.

Transportation

Transportation for the evacuation of health care facilities patients/residents and accompanying staff during an evacuation is a resource-intensive undertaking. Many impaired and incapacitated patients/residents cannot travel on a standard bus or van.

While some patients/residents may travel safely in vans or buses, wheelchair lifts for these vehicles are almost always needed, and some patients/residents undergoing rehabilitation or suffering from debilitating illnesses may require ambulance transport. Consider evacuation at night when there is less disruption with meals and medications. Night transport has worked well in Florida for older patients.

Whichever form of evacuation transportation is required, acquiring and maintaining it on a year-round basis is expensive. The transportation problem has been made worse because the National Disaster Medical System (NDMS) does not support the evacuation of long-term care patients, although this federal policy may be changing. States have initiated ambulance deployment strategies to support evacuation of health care facilities. In addition, there is a national ambulance deployment contract that FEMA has put into place since the 2005 Hurricanes. As of October 1, 2009, the 48 contiguous United States are divided into four FEMA zones. Maximum deployment in a single FEMA zone includes 300 ground ambulances, 25 air ambulances and enough paratransit vehicles to transport 3,500 people. Additional info can be accessed at: www.nasemso.org/Projects/DomesticPreparedness/document/AMR-FEMAcontractoverview2010-10-054page.pdf.

However, the number of available ground transport vehicles in any region is likely insufficient to meet the transport demand created by a massive-scale mass evacuation.

▸ Access to evacuation transportation requires the leverage of multiple systems and careful coordination to prioritize and assign resources. Emergency Operations Centers are tasked with coordination of available transportation resources to support evacuation of health care facilities, including for nursing homes.

▸ School buses are not the panacea for evacuations. School districts differ from state to state and also within states as to ownership and maintenance. In North Carolina, the state owns all of the school buses and has the ability to move these resources across county lines. In other states, some district policies do not allow for cross-county travel, and some narrowly define eligible drivers. Texas reported that school districts there are being advised by their attorneys not to contract with nursing homes due to liability concerns. Even with policy issues resolved, the lack of wheelchair accessibility is a barrier to the use of standard school buses to transport frail patients/ residents.

▸ Recognize the limits of transportation alternatives at the community level.

▸ Advocate for NHs to receive advance notice of mandatory evacuations and state police escorts. Some states' advocates are pushing for advance notice of mandatory evacuations so that they can move frail patients/residents before the roads become clogged. However, a major problem is the uncertainty of actual landfall of a storm when a facility is evacuated too early, e.g., 96 hours prior to an expected landfall.

▸ Include long-term care facilities in state/regional/national transportation planning efforts.

Power Restoration

Hospitals receive priority status for power restoration as they have heavier power dependency needs for their patients, but even with backup generators, fuel can be an issue. Sub-acute hospitals, rehabilitation centers and long-term care facilities, especially those with acute care units have installed generators to support power needs. Communication with the local EOC about their capabilities is critical as part of emergency planning.

The priority status of non-hospital health care facilities for power restoration varies from state to state. Those with an LTC seat at the emergency operations center do seem to have an advantage in advocating for these facilities to be included on the critical infrastructure list.

▸ Educate emergency managers of the similarities between hospital and nursing home populations. Not all emergency managers will be aware of the high-risk health status of today's nursing home resident. Take time to help them to understand that the patient population is similar in many ways to hospital populations. This understanding will help to ensure that nursing homes are viewed as part of the critical infrastructure for power restoration.

▸ Develop a positive and strong relationship with each major power company's disaster response team leader in your state. It is imperative that the nursing home association representative establish a positive relationship with the energy disaster response team leaders. Create a post-disaster communication network to keep them informed of the status of nursing homes in the disaster area and to exchange, in real time, both the status of power restoration, as well as the status of nursing homes needing power restored. The energy responders will come to count on your expertise to help them identify which facilities should go off-line and which can be restored.

▸ Use of generators takes pre-planning. Generator back-up systems need to be checked regularly and have sufficient fuel for four to five days or more. Make sure generator fuel is secure and safe from unauthorized use. Generators for NHs are not "off the shelf." They are designed to accommodate the facility's particular power load, as determined by an electrician. Also, capital improvements that affect power usage have to be factored in, if added since the last generator power assessment. Also, governmental permitting processes and policies for nursing homes acquiring diesel and bio-fuel generators should be expedited. A Florida delegate reported that it takes months to obtain the permits needed for generator systems that use diesel and bio-fuel.

The six hospitals in Brevard County met with their power provider and an agreement is in place that they are the first to be restored to the box after a catastrophic outage such as that following a direct-hit hurricane.

At-Home and Special Needs Patients

Some of the most vulnerable members of society, especially during an emergency, are at-home and special needs patients. Provision needs to be made in emergency planning to protect them and remove them to safety if warranted.

People with Disabilities

Three months after terrorist attacks redefined American life, most of the country's 54 million citizens with disabilities said that they did not feel sufficiently prepared for future crises. According to Harris Interactive survey results released by The National Organization on Disability (N.O.D.):

▸ Fifty-eight percent of people with disabilities say they do not know who to contact about emergency plans for their community in the event of a terrorist attack or other crisis.

▸ Sixty-one percent say that they have not made plans to evacuate their homes quickly and safely.

▸ Among those who are employed full- or part-time, 50 percent say that no plans have been made to evacuate their workplace safely.

"The country as a whole has some catching up to do to be prepared, but these statistics show that people with disabilities lag behind everyone else. This is a critical discrepancy, because those of us with disabilities must in fact be better prepared so we are not at a disadvantage in an emergency," said N.O.D. President Alan A. Reich. "It is critical that all plans for emergency preparedness consider the special needs of people with disabilities. We strongly advocate that individuals with disabilities themselves be included in the planning process at all levels."

These people need to be even more prepared than the average citizen. See the State of Florida report from "Disaster and Emergency Preparedness Report of the 2008 Regional Survey of Persons with Disabilities Phase 3 July 2008."

First Responders

> It is incumbent on first responders to learn how best to perform a rescue using equipment and procedures that facilitate safe evacuation for any person with a disability.

People with disabilities are entitled to the same level of protection in an emergency as everyone else – no more, no less. The "reasonable accommodation" mandated in the Americans with Disabilities Act (ADA) is intended to provide the same level of safety and utility for people with disabilities as is provided to everyone. Key points to consider are as follows:

▸ Remember that a person with a disability has unique abilities and limitations. Accommodations should be made that emphasize their abilities.

- Include the person in the decision-making process when selecting special equipment and design of procedures.

- Familiarize yourself with the building and occupants in your response area; identify coworkers, neighbors and friends who can be of assistance in an emergency.

- Participate in the development of emergency evacuation planning for the occupancies in your community before the emergencies occur.

People with disabilities are increasingly moving into the mainstream of society, which contributes to the diversity that has been this country's strength. Further, we cannot predict when anyone of us may need assistance, such as in the case of a broken leg or the development of heart or lung disease.

Questions to Ask

☐ Does your Local Emergency Planning Committee (LEPC) include individuals with disabilities as active members?

☐ Do your Emergency Operation Plans (EOP) take into consideration individuals' capability to evacuate with little or no assistance?

☐ Have members of your fire or emergency services department had awareness training in evacuating people with disabilities?

☐ Do you have a seat at the EOC and, more specifically, at the ESF 8 desk?

Identifying Those with Special Needs

First responders need to take into consideration that there are many individuals who are protective of their right to independence and privacy and who may be reluctant to be identified. In the development of plans, think of each individual as one who happens to have a particular disability. Do not make the mistake of lumping together all persons with disabilities into one group or category. For example, there are building emergency evacuation plans and codes on which they were based, containing instructions for all persons with disabilities to go to an area of refuge and wait for members of the emergency team to escort them to safety. As a general rule, there is no reason that a person who is blind or deaf cannot use the stairs to make an independent escape, as long as he or she can effectively be notified of the need to evacuate and can find the stairway.

You must take into consideration legal and security issues, as well. For instance, have you a policy about admitting sex offenders to public shelters or people on probation or parole?

Locating People with Disabilities in Your Community to Include in Emergency Preparedness Planning

- Contact local agencies and organizations that support persons with disabilities.

- Contact your State Vocational and Rehabilitation Agency. Part of their work is to introduce volunteer and public service organizations to their clients.

  ▷ View the Federal Consumer Information Center's online list of State Vocational and Rehabilitation Agencies.

- ▷ Search the Internet using a phrase such as "[your state] Vocational Rehabilitation."
  - ▷ Look in the government pages of your local phone book for state or local listings such as "Rehabilitation Services Administration" or "Rehabilitation Information."
- ▸ There are several hundred Centers for Independent Living (CIL) across the country.
  - ▷ CILs are community-based resource and advocacy centers managed by and for people with disabilities, promoting independent living and equal access for all persons with physical, mental, cognitive and sensory disabilities.
- ▸ Contact your state or local government's committee, commission or council on disabilities. These are often part of the governor's office or cabinet.
- ▸ Contact your state's Department of Veterans Affairs facilities, which serve people with disabilities.
- ▸ Contact your local ADA coordinator, who usually can be located through the Mayor's office or county government office.
- ▸ Contact local church congregations, which may be aware of specific community members with disabilities.
- ▸ Ask professionals who serve people with disabilities, such as special education teachers, or occupational, physical, or speech therapists, if they can suggest individuals to participate in emergency planning. You might try contacting the National Rehabilitation Association.
- ▸ Many hospitals have home health agencies that support persons with newly diagnosed illnesses or injuries that result in functional access or mobility needs. Home health encourages emergency planning of family members or caregivers assisting such persons, to prepare to shelter in place, register in general or special needs shelters if needed, or plan to evacuate an area ahead of an event. Home Health also conducts planning to maintain contact with their clientele through phone contact and visits, as appropriate, during emergencies and disasters.

Vision (Blind or Low Vision)

When you approach a person who has vision impairments, announce your presence. Speak naturally and directly to the individual not through a third party. Say something like, "Hi, I am Firefighter Jones." Describe the action to be taken, and then ask the person to tell you the best way to assist him or her.

First responders should take steps to ensure that after exiting the building, individuals with impaired vision are not abandoned but are led to a place of safety. Someone should remain with them until the emergency is over. There is no need to speak louder to persons with visual impairments.

Florida has recently developed a course to assist emergency response staff to support persons with disabilities. Arrangements are underway to place this course on the American Red Cross and FEMA Websites.

Tips for Assisting People with Visual Impairments

▸ It's OK to use words such as "see," "look" or "blind." Let the individual grasp your arm or shoulder lightly for guidance. He or she may choose to walk slightly behind you to gauge your body reactions to obstacles.

▸ It is helpful to use clock settings to describe the location of objects or even food on a plate (meat is at 6 o'clock position; potatoes are at 10 o'clock and peas are at 2 o'clock).

▸ Be sure to mention stairs, doorways, narrow passages and ramps.

▸ When guiding to a seat, place the person's hand on the back of the chair.

▸ If leading several individuals at the same time, ask them to hold each other's arms.

Dog Guides

Traditionally, the term "service animal" referred to seeing-eye dogs© for people with vision impairments. However, today there are many other types of "service animals." In addition to guide dogs for the blind, there are:

▸ Hearing dogs for people who are deaf

▸ Seizure dogs for people who have seizure disorders

▸ Assist animals for people with motor impairments

▸ Companion animals for people with psychiatric impairments

Tips for Assisting Owners with Service Dogs

▸ Do not pet or offer the dog food without the permission of the owner.

▸ When the dog is wearing its harness, it is on duty. In the event you are asked to take the dog while assisting the individual, it is recommended that you hold the leash and not the dog's harness.

▸ Plan for the dog to be evacuated with the owner.

Service Animals

As of March 15, 2011, only "dogs" are recognized as "service animals" under Titles II and III of the ADA. Service dogs are working animals, not pets. The work or task a service dog has been trained to provide must be directly related to the person's disability. Dogs whose sole function is to provide comfort or emotional support don't qualify as "service dogs" under the ADA's rules. Service animals are working animals, not pets. Examples of such work or tasks include: guiding people who are blind, alerting people who are deaf, pulling a wheelchair, alerting and protecting a person who is having a seizure, reminding a person with mental illness to take prescribed medications, calming a person with Post-Traumatic Stress Disorder (PTSD) during an anxiety attack, or performing other tasks or duties.

Generally, Title II and III entities must permit service dogs to accompany people with disabilities in all areas where members of the public are allowed. For example, in a hospital it would be inappropriate to exclude a service dogs from areas such as patient rooms, clinics, cafeterias or examination rooms. However, it may be appropriate to exclude a service dog from Operating Rooms or Burn Units, where the animal's presence may compromise a sterile environment.

When it isn't obvious what service an animal provides, only limited inquiries are allowed. Staff may ask two questions:

▸ Is the dog a service animal required because of a disability?

▸ What work or task has the dog been trained to perform on behalf of the disabled person?

Staff members are not allowed to:

▸ Ask about the person's disability.

▸ Require medical documentation, or require a special identification card or training documentation for the dog.

▸ Ask that the dog demonstrate its ability to perform the work or task.

Hearing Impairments (Deaf or Hard of Hearing)

Hearing impairments range from mild hearing loss to an extreme or profound deafness, the level at which an individual receives no benefit from aural input. Many persons who are hearing impaired can use their residual hearing effectively with assistance from hearing aids or other sound amplification devices, often augmented by lip reading. However, hearing aids also amplify background sounds. For example, the sound of emergency alarms interferes with or even drowns out voice announcements, rendering the emergency voice communication system useless. An accommodation for this problem is to provide individuals with a tactile/vibratory pager, which is tied into the building fire notification system.

When the audible alarm is activated, they are simultaneously notified by the vibration of the pager.

Another major problem of emergency notification faced by persons who are deaf or hard of hearing is that they cannot keep up with storm warnings on radio and television. In Florida, TV stations now close-caption their hurricane coverage and several deaf organizations have set up TDD/TTY hotlines to keep persons up-to-date on storm warnings and evacuation orders.

When approaching a person who is deaf or hard of hearing, and the person does not have visual contact with you, e.g., if you are entering a room, flick the lights on and off to draw attention to your presence.

If you are rescuing a person who is deaf or hard of hearing, do not allow others to interrupt or joke with you while conveying the emergency information. Be patient; the individual may have difficulty comprehending the urgency of your message.

Tips for Assisting People with Hearing Impairments

▸ Face the light. Do not cover or turn your face away, and never chew gum.

▸ Establish eye contact with the person, even if an interpreter is present.

- Use facial expressions and hand gestures as visual cues.

- Check to see if you have been understood and repeat, if necessary.

- Offer pencil and paper. Write slowly, and let the individual read as you write. Written communication may be especially important if you are unable to understand the individual's speech.

- Provide the individual with a flashlight for signaling his or her location, in the event that he or she is separated from the rescuing team or buddy, and to facilitate lip-reading in the dark.

Cognitive Impairments

People with developmental disabilities may experience limitation with cognitive abilities, motor abilities and social abilities. The individual may have difficulty in recognizing rescuers or being motivated to act in an emergency. These individuals may also have difficulty in responding to instructions which involve more than a small number of simple actions. Keep in mind that:

- Visual perception of written instructions or signs may be confused.

- Sense of direction may be limited, requiring someone to accompany them.

- Ability to understand speech is often more developed than his or her own vocabulary.

- The individual should be treated as an adult who happens to have a cognitive or learning disability.

Tips for Assisting People with Cognitive Impairments

- Be patient.

- Break down information into simple steps.

- Use simple signals or symbols.

- Do not talk about a person to others in front of him or her.

- Do not talk down to or treat the person as a child.

- Provide pictures, symbols or diagrams instead of words.

- Read written information.

- Provide written information on audiotape.

- Use voice output on the computer.

- Use Reading Pen for single words.

- Use line guide to identify or highlight one line of text at a time.

Use of Pictures to Replace Spoken Language

You can use picture (communication) boards to replace the spoken language. The boards have pictures of different parts of the body that can be pointed at to identify the location of the problem. It also contains pictures of different complaints – stomach ache, ear ache, burns, bites, etc., which can be used to identify the cause of the problem.

Care-Receiver

This communication board is to be used to assist you in expressing your needs in times of disaster or other emergency situations. If you are the victim of such circumstances and are having problems expressing your needs, simply point to the picture or phrase that represents your situation or identify an item you need.

Caregiver

This communication board has been designed to bridge communication gaps in times of disaster or other emergency situations. The gaps may result from language barriers, disability, age, or the trauma and confusion associated with the event. As a result, critical information could be difficult to exchange. By either acknowledging or pointing to the appropriate picture, you can better assess health conditions.

Wheelchair Users

Because people who use wheelchairs have a wide variety of abilities and limitations, it is difficult to generalize their needs. Following are some useful questions to consider in understanding common limitations.

▸ Is the person able to stand or walk without the aid of the wheelchair?

▸ If yes, how long can the person stand or walk unaided?

▸ Does the person have full, partial, or no use of the upper extremities?

Wheelchair users are trained in special techniques to transfer from one chair to another. Depending on their upper body strength, they may be able to do much of the work themselves. As with persons with vision impairments, ask first what you can do to help them. During rescues in which the person is transferred from his or her wheelchair into an evacuation chair, the first responder needs to consider that once the person has been taken to a place of safety, the wheelchair should be waiting for him or her, if possible. People who depend on their wheelchairs for mobility have expressed concern about their wheelchairs being left behind.

Ask the person what would be the best way to assist them. They will tell you. The recommended patient carries can be safely used to avoid injury to patients, if used correctly. Staff needs to be trained in such methods with regular exercises.

Tips for Assisting Wheelchair Users

▸ When giving directions to a person in a wheelchair, consider distance, weather conditions and physical obstacles such as stairs, curbs and steep hills.

▸ Relax and speak naturally. Do not be embarrassed if you happen to use accepted common expressions, such as "got to be running along," that seem to relate to the person's disability.

▸ When addressing a person who uses a wheelchair, do not lean on the wheelchair unless you have permission to do so. A wheelchair is part of an individual's personal space.

▸ When talking to a person who uses a wheelchair, look at and speak directly to that person, rather than through a companion.

▸ When talking with a person in a wheelchair for more than a few minutes, use a chair whenever possible. This can facilitate conversation.

▸ Terms, such as "wheelchair bound" or "confined to a wheelchair," are inappropriate. Using a wheelchair does not mean confinement.

▸ When greeting a person who uses a wheelchair, it is appropriate to offer to shake hands with that person, even if he or she has upper extremity limitations.

Mobility

Non-Ambulatory Patients

Wheeled Beds: From a hazardous room or location, this is slow. Gurneys or wheelchairs can also be used.

Blanket Litters: May be used if stored poles are available (fold in thirds) or if edges are rolled.

Blanket Carry: Patient behind and facing you, blanket under patient's arms and over your shoulder, knot held in front of you. Blanket should be folded diagonally. Lean forward to carry.

Blanket Drag: Patient diagonal, lift at head and pull head first, even down stairs.

Cradle Drop (patient same size or smaller than rescuer): Lock the wheels on the bed. Double a blanket lengthwise and place it on the floor parallel to the bed. If approaching from the patient's right side, slip your left arm under the patient's neck, grasp the left shoulder in your left hand, slip your right arm under the knees and grasp them with your right hand. Your right knee or thigh, depending on the height of the bed, is placed against the bed and opposite the patient's thigh. Both feet are flat on the floor about six inches apart, with the left foot about six inches from the bed. If the patient is approached from the left side, the procedure is reversed. The patient is pulled from the bed. No lifting is necessary. Pull with both hands and push with your right knee or thigh. The moment that the patient starts to leave the bed, drop onto your left knee. When the patient is clear of the bed, your extended right knee supports the patient's knees and your left arm supports the head and shoulders. The cradle formed by the knee and arm protects the back. The patient slides gently to the blanket, and the blanket is pulled from the room, head first. The relative position of the patient's body is important as you cannot maintain the balance necessary if you pull the patient's buttocks instead of the knees or thigh out onto your knee. This removal is for patients too heavy for one associate to carry, for low beds, and for bed and oxygen tent fires.

Kneel Drop: The kneel drop is a variation of the basic cradle drop. The blanket is doubled lengthwise and placed on the floor parallel to the bed. Approaching the patient from the patient's left, slip your right arm under the patient's neck and grasp the right shoulder in your right hand. Place your left knee or thigh, depending on the height of the bed, against the bed and opposite the patient's thigh. Both of your feet should be flat on the floor about six inches apart with the right foot about six inches from the bed. No lifting is necessary. Pull with both hands and push with the left knee or thigh. The very moment that the patient starts to leave the bed, drop onto your right knee. When the patient is clear of the bed, drop your left knee beside the right knee, lean forward with your back straight and let the patient slide down your body onto your knees. In other words, pull the patient out onto your chest and not out on the knees. Draw your knees from under the patient's body and pull the patient from the room. This removal is particularly useful for handling excessive weight, fracture, post-op and pregnancy cases, when only one rescuer is available. If the patient is lying in fire, the cradle drop or kneel drop will ensure the least involvement of the rescuer.

Semi and Ambulatory Patients

Extremity Carry (Two Rescuers): Approaching from the patient's left, the first rescuer, standing with feet together, slips her right arm under the patient's upper left arm. Bring the patient to a sitting position by taking one step with the left foot towards the foot of the bed. This move employs the swing of your whole body. You can gain additional leverage if you push your right shoulder against the patient's left shoulder once the patient is in motion. When the patient is sitting, the second rescuer grasps the ankles and swings the patient's feet off the bed. If the patient is approached from the right, all the mechanics are reversed. When the patient is sitting, the first rescuer places her arms through the armpits and grips her own wrists above the patient's chest. The second rescuer approaches from the same side and halts at the patient's feet. With her left hand under the patient's right heel, the second rescuer then pulls the right ankle clear of the bed as she slides between the patient's legs as far as the patient's right knee. As the second rescuer makes a half turn left, she grasps the patient's right knee under her arm. Completing the turn, she transfers her left hand to the patient's left knee which she then encircles with her left arm. She now has a leg under each arm. Both rescuers then take one step away from the bed and carry the patient from the room. Like so many other carries, this involves a "hugging" action, with the patient's back carried tight against the first rescuer's chest and the patient's shoulder as close to the level of hers as possible. To unload the patient in the corridor, the second rescuer stoops with her right foot slightly behind and about six inches from her left lowering the patient's legs to the floor. The first rescuer lets the patient slide down her body until the buttocks reach the floor. Then, she lowers the patient to his back. This is very useful when the path of exit is narrow because of furniture or fire.

Pack Strap: With the patient behind and facing you, and his arms over your shoulders crossed in front of you, grasp each of his wrists with your opposite hand. Lean forward to carry.

Hip Carry: Sit on the bed as the patient faces you lying on his side. Reach behind his back to grasp his armpit while your other arm reaches around to grasp his knees. Lean forward to carry across your hips.

Swing Method: With one carrier on each side of the patient, grasp each other's wrist under the patient's knees and each other's shoulder behind the patient's back (under his arms). This is especially used for seated patients.

Three Carriers: With all on one side of the patient, lift and roll the patient to face your chest. Carry feet first. This can be aided by a fourth carrier, lifting from the other side till weight is up and balanced.

Six Carriers: With three on each side of the patient, full spine is supported by alternating arms underneath.

Ambulant with Assistance

Someone using a walking aide, such as a crutch or a cane, might be able to negotiate stairs independently. One hand is used to grasp the handrail, while the other hand is used for the crutch or cane. Here, it is best not to interfere with this person's movement. You might be of assistance by offering to carry the extra crutch. Also, if the stairs are crowded, you can act as a buffer and run interference.

The Cradle Carry method is normally used for non-ambulatory patients but can be used for ambulatory patients who need assistance. It is used when the person has little or no arm strength. It is safest if the person being carried weighs less than the carrier's weight. The choice of a particular carry has little to do with the disability of the person to be rescued, and more to do with his or her size, abilities and certain problems, such as leg spasms.

The choice between the carries relates then to the general physical attributes of both the rescuer and the rescuee. As the size of the rescuee approaches the size of the rescuer, the difficulty of choosing a technique increases and becomes more and more dependent on the abilities of the rescuee.

Swing- or Chair-Carry: The advantage of the Swing- or Chair-Carry is that partners can support, with practice and coordination, a person whose weight is the same or even greater than their own weight. The disadvantage is increased awkwardness in vertical travel (stair descent) due to the complexity of the two-person carry. Also, three persons abreast may exceed the effective width of the stairway. Stand on opposite sides of the individual being rescued. Take the rescuee's arm on your side and place it around your shoulder. Grasp your carry partner's forearm behind the rescuee, at the small of his or her back. Reach under the rescuee's knees and grasp your carry partner's other wrist. Lean in close to the individual and lift at the count of three. Continue pressing into the individual being carried to provide additional support. After completion of the lift, shift the rescuee upward for a more comfortable carry.

Mobility - In-Chair Carry: The wheelchair user is anxious to be returned to his or her wheelchair after the rescue; therefore, the in-chair evacuation is desirable when feasible.

One-Person Assist:

‣ Grasp the pushing grips, if the wheelchair has them.
‣ Stand one step above and behind the wheelchair.
‣ Tilt the wheelchair backward until a balance (fulcrum) is achieved.
‣ Keep your center of gravity low.
‣ Descend frontward.

▸ Let the back wheels gradually lower to the next step.

▸ If possible, have another person assist you.

Two-Person Assist: Positioning of second rescuer:

▸ Stand in front of the wheelchair.

▸ Face the wheelchair.

▸ Stand one, two or three steps down (dependent on the height of the rescuer).

▸ Grasp the frame of the wheelchair.

▸ Push into the wheelchair.

▸ Descend stairs backward.

The person in front should be careful not to lift the wheelchair, as this places additional weight on the person assisting behind the wheelchair. Tilt backward until a balance (fulcrum) is achieved.

Three-Person Assist: Position for second and third rescuers:

▸ Face direction of descent.

▸ Flank the wheelchair.

▸ Stay in line with the two front (smaller) wheels.

▸ Stand one step/tread lower than rescuer behind wheelchair.

▸ Grasp the frame of the wheelchair.

▸ Push into the wheelchair.

Helpless patients may be rolled in a blanket and dragged to a safe location. Disoriented patients (e.g., Psych) should be handled like other patients. If time and circumstances permit, alternate the confused ambulatory patients between coherent patients.

Evacuation Devices

There are a large number of devices that can assist in an evacuation – from chairs to sleds. They are all designed to protect the patient while being moved and most can be handled by one member of staff irrespective of the weight of the patient.

There are evacu-sleds that cocoon the patient and mattress together, allowing medical personnel to move patients along hallways and downstairs without injury. The Missouri Hospital Association has utilized Med Sleds which allow a 250-pound patient to be lifted by a 120-pound staff member. The devices are lightweight, compact and easy to store and are able to carry oxygen, IV bags and other medical devices. The Evacupod is an inflatable device that allows the patient to be strapped in securely, and then moved safely. It is important to assess your own needs and requirements and to have all necessary equipment available with people trained to use it.

Case Study

When the first plane hit the twin towers on September 11, 2001, John Abruzzo, like others, rushed to the stairwell. However, evacuation for John would prove to be much more difficult than others, as he is a C 5-6 quadriplegic who relies on an electric wheelchair for mobility. With use of the emergency evacuation chair, John was able to make an escape to safety. "It took us an hour and a half to get down 69 floors." In the first attack on the World Trade Center in February 1993, John's evacuation took six hours, during which he was carried in his electric chair from the 69th floor to the 44th floor, where he was transferred to a stretcher and taken out of the building.

Shortly after the 1993 bombing, the Port Authority purchased a number of products and systems to aid in the evacuation and life-safety of the World Trade Center occupants. The implementation of these products proved successful on 9/11. Lights stayed on while John and his friends evacuated, ventilation systems in the stairwells minimized smoke infiltration, and the evacuation chairs became a real life-saver. Several other people with disabilities were successfully evacuated with evacuation chairs. John and his group exited the tower and were out of harm's way, just 10 minutes before its collapse.

Patient Critical Evacuation Information Tracking Form

Blank Forms are available online. Please see Table of Contents for instructions.

The following form could potentially be used by a hospital's home health department to be given to their community living clientele who may need to be registered for a special needs shelter.

Sample Voluntary Registration Request for Medically Fragile Individuals

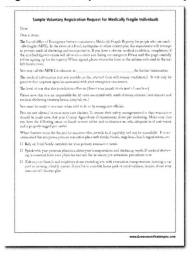

Blank Forms are available online. Please see Table of Contents for instructions.

Emergency Operations Plans must cover every conceivable eventuality. Planners must hope for the best but plan for the worst. If planners work on the theory "it won't happen to us", they are heading for an even greater disaster.

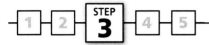

STEP 3
Evacuation Planning

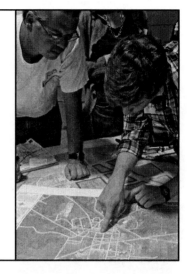

Evacuation: Evacuation of patients is a measure of last resort, but is occasionally necessary, especially in extreme situations. Many different conditions or vulnerabilities already mentioned can cause the evacuation of a hospital, but the process of evacuation itself can also be vulnerable to disruption that can seriously aggravate the health and safety of patients. Frequently, a flood, earthquake or a windstorm can cause blockage of access roads, cutting off a hospital from normal evacuation routes, as happened during Hurricane Katrina. Surface escape routes were under water and unusable; and even air evacuation was impaired because many ground-level helicopter landing pads were under water. Elevated helipads located on roof tops or elevated parking structures proved invaluable features in this type of an emergency. The spatial relationship to the hospital building was another aspect that greatly influenced the evacuation and reduced the risk of aggravating patients' condition. Helipads physically connected to the hospital were most useful, because patients could be transported directly and very rapidly from the upper levels of the hospital to the helipad without interference from other hospital functions.

The following are examples of what could lead to activation of any given hospital's evacuation plan:

Internal Emergencies

Fire, smoke, hazardous materials release or irritant fumes in the following areas:

- Laboratories
- Mechanical rooms
- Operating rooms
- Emergency department

- Clinics and patient rooms
- Facility services and maintenance areas

Loss of environmental support services

- Heat
- Water supply
- Air conditioning
- Sterilization
- Electrical power
- Computer network
- Telecommunications (paging, telephones)

Loss of medical gases

- Oxygen
- Compressed air
- Vacuum suction
- Other examples
- Explosion or bomb threat
- Police actions
- Armed or violent visitor

External Emergencies

Natural Hazards

- Earthquake
- Hurricane
- Flood
- Tornado
- Blizzard

Other Hazards

- Regional power outage
- Civil disturbance
- Terrorism
- Transportation accidents
- Hazardous materials releases

▸ Contaminated victims/toxic agents

▸ Radiation

General Planning Notes

There are times when a facility must be evacuated for an extended period of time because the structure is unsafe. Depending on the circumstances, there may be one or more similar facilities in your area that are not affected by the same event. Therefore, the following information is provided to assist you in caring for your residents/patients during major emergencies/disasters.

 Must Do ——————————

It is recommended that each facility manager meet with the managers of other similar facility managers in his/her area and develop a Memorandum of Understanding/Agreement.

The purpose of such an agreement is to form pairings of similar facilities. If your facility must be evacuated, your residents are moved to another similar facility until your facility can be occupied. It is the facility owner's/manager's responsibility to ensure procedures and applicable agreements are in place to move his/her residents/patients to safety. Any size facility should have clearly defined roles and responsibilities assigned to staff. Core Competencies can be assigned to each level of response. Florida Department of Health's version can be accessed at: www.doh.state.fl.us/demo/BPR/PDFs/CoreCompetenciesUpdatedSpring2011.pdf.

Maps, floor plans, personnel rosters, etc., should be added to the applicable Annex as Appendices. It is important that larger facilities develop an alerting or call-out roster for each Annex. The Staff Functions by Department and Job Assignment section of each Annex will aid you in developing an alerting or call-out roster.

Disaster Emergency Planning

Readiness for facility evacuation requires several stages of preparation and implementation. The entire process of assessing a facility's readiness to evacuate can be established by:

▸ Defining the authorities for evacuation in the community

▸ Defining a facility's legal responsibility and role regarding evacuation

▸ Assessing hazards and identifying risks that might require or complicate evacuation of a facility

▸ Developing strategies for evacuation of the facility, or supporting facilities that evacuate to a host facility

▸ Developing and implementing an evacuation/sheltering plan, operational procedures, training programs and drills

▸ Continual reevaluation of plan and procedures based upon drills and actual evacuations.

Defining Authorities and Responsibilities

The authorities and legal responsibility for evacuation provide documentation and guidance for understanding evacuation directions in the community.

Planning

The vast majority of hospitals have evacuation plans in place that deal with the most common evacuation they face, fire. However, fire plans are not comprehensive and do not address all of the issues.

▸ Fire evacuation plans are written to effect rapid evacuation of the affected area, as patients are routinely incapable of self-preservation, but these plans rarely address a full facility evacuation that may be necessary over time (several hours to several days).

▸ Drills of the Fire Evacuation plan are routinely conducted but seldom include the actual evacuation of the area; therefore, the plan is never stressed to see if it actually works.

▸ Because these plans deal with one reason for the evacuation, fire, vulnerability analyses performed have not included other pertinent issues, such as:

  ▹ Location and vulnerability of generators (flooding)

  ▹ Ability to evacuate from roof

  ▹ Equipment necessary to move patients

  ▹ Staging areas

  ▹ Transportation to other facilities

  ▹ Transportation resources: hospital often use the same non-emergency ambulance companies

  ▹ Routes: what routes will the transportation take, remembering that roads will be busy.

Evacuation plans should be written to encompass all gradations of an evacuation, from the "shelter–in-place" scenario up to and including a full-scale hospital evacuation.

Scope of Evacuations

Evacuation planning must be done keeping in mind that the scope of the evacuation can grow over time depending on the nature of the event. In fact, an evacuation can start as a "shelter-in-place" scenario, where minor adjustments are made to accommodate the event, but essentially no one is moved. The "shelter-in-place" strategy can move over the course of several hours or days to a full-scale campus evacuation, where the entire hospital, its patients and staff must be relocated.

Examples of escalating scope of evacuations:

▸ Defend in place

▸ Single department/floor/unit

▸ Section – Multiple floors/units within a single building

▸ Entire building to another location on campus

- ▸ Entire campus evacuation
- ▸ Citywide evacuation

In addition, the timeframe around evacuations can be different, ranging from a rapid evacuation in the case where the event is life threatening to a slow growing need to evacuate as was the case in New Orleans during Hurricane Katrina.

Types of Evacuations

Traditionally hospitals have focused on horizontal and vertical evacuations – Horizontally moving to a safer location on the same floor, or vertically (up or down) to another floor that is unaffected by the event. Hospitals now need to put in place planning that encompasses moving patients/staff and others to a safe haven/staging area in preparation for a move to another facility.

Creating Comprehensive Evacuation Plans

In order to address the full scope of the stages of evacuations, it is necessary to put together plans that address three basic elements:

- ▸ Facility Issues
- ▸ People Issues
- ▸ Support Services Issues

Additionally, it is important to understand that these plans are designed so that the hospital utilizing them can scale the evacuation to their individual needs and recognize the fact that the process of evacuation may escalate over the course of several hours to several days, from clearing several floors to a full campus evacuation.

Facility Issues

Evacuation plans need to include tools that allow the HEICS team – and, in particular, the Incident Commander – the ability to identify rapidly areas of the hospital that require a high priority for evacuation, areas of vulnerability and areas that have potential risk.

Drilling down details building by building, and then floor by floor within buildings, is necessary to get to the specific details of the evacuation itself. Identification of staging areas where patients will be sent temporarily should be identified early on so that routes to safe havens can be incorporated into the specific departmental evacuation plans. In addition, hospitals must work with their Engineering and Facility Departments to evaluate the feasibility of evacuation of patients from a rooftop. Structurally, many buildings cannot support the weight of a helicopter; therefore, it is necessary to determine if this is a feasible evacuation route.

📋 Checklist

Evacuation Tool Kit

☐ Laminated Evacuation Triage levels

☐ Pre-Strung Fluorescent Tags, if needed

☐ Removable Labels - identifies areas that have been checked and evacuated

☐ Permanent Markers

☐ Rubber Bands for Medical Records if electronic medical records are not available

☐ Patient Tracking Tools

☐ Staff Tracking Tools

☐ Visitor Tracking Tools

☐ Patient Critical Evacuation Information Form

☐ Sheet Protectors for Transfer Documentation to Accompany Patient

☐ Non-Skid Socks for Ambulatory Patients without Shoes

☐ Wind Up Flashlight

☐ Fluorescent Vest

Comprehensive Layout of the Hospital Campus

The easiest way to obtain a high level look at the entire hospital campus is by utilizing a simple stacking diagram. These can be easily created in either excel or word. The stacking diagram will give a floor by floor view of:

▸ Patient care areas

▸ Critical patient care area

▸ Non patient areas

▸ Vacant space

These areas can be coded using a gray-scale coloring scheme, so that plans can be easily and quickly reproduced and distributed during the event. Symbols should be used to identify areas that contain hazardous chemicals or materials, as well as those floors that may have connecting bridges between buildings. You can also use life-safety drawings for SWAT.

Stacking Diagram

KEY

| PATIENT CARE AREA |
| CRITICAL CARE PATIENT AREA |
| NON PATIENT CARE AREA |
| VACANT |

ROOF	ROOF
RESEARCH	NURSING UNIT MED SURG
NURSING UNIT MED SURG	NURSING UNIT SURGICAL
CLOSED NURSING UNIT	NURSING UNIT CARDIAC
NURSING UNIT MEDICINE	NURSING UNIT ICU
NURSING UNIT MEDICINE	NURSING UNIT ICU
NURSING UNIT PEDIATRICS	MECHANICAL ROOM
NURSING UNIT	OR LOCKERS/FAN ROOM
OPERATING ROOMS/PACU	CYSTO/AMB SURG
CENTRAL STERILE	MAT MGT/PHARMACY
CAFETERIA/ DINING ROOM TRANSPORTATION OFFICE/ FOOD SERVICE OFFICE	LOBBY/ADMITTING PAT MEDICIAID OFFICE UM ADMINISTRATION
KITCHEN	KITCHEN
BUILDING 1	**BUILDING 2**

		ROOF
		MACHINE ROOM
ROOF		RESEARCH
MACHINE ROOM		RESEARCH
MACHINE ROOM	ROOF	RESEARCH
ANIMAL RESEARCH	MACHINE ROOM	RESEARCH
NURSING UNIT PSYCH	ON CALL ROOMS	RESEARCH
NURSING UNIT PSYCH	LABS	RESEARCH
MEDICINE ADMIN	ADMINISTRA-TION	BIOMED
NURSING UNTI MED/SURG	NURSING UNIT REHAB	OUTPATIENT REHAB
NURSING UNIT MED/SURG	VACANT	NUC. MED/NUC CARDIOLOGY
LABS	ENDOSCOPY	LABS/EKG
RADIOLOGY	ULTRASOUND	CATH LAB/EPS
OUTPATIENT CLINICS	OUTPATIENT CLINICS	MEDICAL RECORDS
EMERGENCY DEPARTMENT	EMERGENCY DEPT	MRI/ SECURITY
MACHINE ROOM	MACHINE ROOM	MACHINE ROOM
BUILDING 3	**BUILDING 4**	**BUILDING 5**

Hazardous Chemicals Present

Connecting Bridges

This stacking diagram is also used to illustrate where fire drills are completed and adjacent smoke departments.

Building Directory:

A building directory will provide details of each department, service and/or administrative offices that are on each individual floor of the building. This is critical in understanding priority for evacuation, as well as for assurance that all staff, patients and others have been accounted for. It is recommended that when gathering this data, the main evacuation routes should also be identified to assist the Incident Commander and others in understanding how traffic will flow during the evacuation.

Departmental Detail

The next and final level of detail necessary is the departmental level detail. Each service, nursing unit or department should create a departmental evacuation plan using a standard template. The template should be brief and include critical information only. For the purposes of the evacuation, where it is critical that patients be quickly taken out of harm's way, the template concentrates on gathering the patient care information necessary. The recommended template includes:

▸ Department/Unit/Service type

▸ Number and type of beds

▸ Specialized medical equipment

▸ Presence and type of hazardous chemicals

▸ Locked or open unit

▸ Presence and type of medical gases

▸ Location of fire exits

▸ Evacuation route

▸ Location of staging area

These templates, once completed, should be kept both in the command center and in the department itself, reviewed and revised annually and shared with staff on an annual basis.

Staging Area

When an evacuation entails a single department/floor or unit, or even multiple floors within a single building, patients should be assigned to vacant beds in other non-affected units within the hospital campus bearing in mind the location of smoke compartments. It is also feasible that patients could be sent to closed units for an interim period until it is deemed safe for the patients to return to their original floors.

In the case where an entire building or entire hospital campus requires evacuation, it is assumed that this will take place over time, and in an orderly fashion, at the direction of the Incident Commander. In this scenario, this plan assumes the following:

▸ The Emergency Department will go on diversion and the inflow of patients will stop. Instead, the ED will begin to function as a dispatcher, if this is where patients are being sent. It may be preferable to use another entrance.

Tip ————————

Staging area(s) should be large enough to support several patients on stretchers and/ or allow set up of cots or air mattresses. If onsite, a discharge area should be designated for patients who are stable enough to discharge home, but are awaiting transportation or family members to pick them up.

The arrangements for transfer for patients to other health care facilities will be the responsibility of the designated person coordinating this directly with the receiving facility in consultation with the local departments of health and other local and state officials. This person is responsible for communicating with external authorities about numbers of persons to be evacuated and how many have been moved as the process continues, number of transportation assets needed and what kind. It might need support from Planning (to support staff traveling with patients), Operations (which patients need transferring, ensuring accepting physicians; this is often the role for Nursing working with the Chief Medical Staff Officer) and the Logistics sections (coordinating supplies to accompany patients transfers).

The physical transfer of the patients, (arrangements for ambulance, ambulette, etc.) will fall under the auspices of the Transportation Unit Leader in consultation with the Office of Emergency Management. These arrangements should already be in place.

‣ A staging area will be utilized as an interim location for inpatients prior to transport to other health care facilities, or prior to discharge if so determined. Patients coming from inpatient units will be transported to the pre-determined staging area and, once there, be re-assessed. Patients will remain in the staging area until such time as transfer has been arranged. At that point, patients will be transported to the Emergency Department where they will be readied for transfer or where you have designated.

Staffing for the staging area should be consistent with the level of acuity on the inpatient units and consist of physicians, registered nurses, nursing assistants and other clerical staff. The Planning Chief would assume the responsibility for staffing this area initially out of the labor pool and/or redeploying staff from the ambulatory setting. As the inpatient units are evacuated, staff from that area will then report to the labor pool for redeployment to the ED or staging area, as necessary. The overall responsibility for the care delivered in the staging area would fall under the responsibility of the Operations Chief under the Medical Care Director. The staff in the staging area will participate in the tracking and reconciliation of patients as they move from point to point.

People Issues

In any evacuation scenario, whether it be a single floor, single building or total hospital campus, assessing, triaging, tracking and reconciling patients, staff, visitors and others as they move throughout the evacuation is the single most important aspect of the plan. You have to detail who is going to inform the patient's family and where calls are forwarded if the hospital has to close.

Clear lines of authority are also necessary to coordinate a systematic and safe evacuation. The use of ICS is imperative to the success of any evacuation. A review of the ICS for hospitals reveals no need to create additional positions; however, each floor or inpatient unit needs to have a person coordinating the evacuation for that area. For the purposes of this document, we will refer to that position as the UNIT EVACUATION LEADER. The Unit Evacuation Leader should be an administrative or operational person, one that is assigned to the area being evacuated by the Incident Commander. This role should not be assumed by clinical staff of that nursing unit, as they will be occupied with triaging and readying patients for transport. HICS designates 52 positions, but many hospitals have consolidated this to around a dozen.

Planning Steps:

▸ System for prioritizing/triaging patients for evacuation

▸ Tagging system to identify levels of care

▸ Identifying and readying patients for evacuation

▸ Medical records

▸ Critical medications

▸ Accounting for patients/families/visitors/staff

▸ System for inventory of patients/staff

▸ System to designate when rooms/floors are empty

▸ Develop an evacuation kit for every area

System for Prioritizing/Triaging and Tagging Inpatients for Evacuation

A systematic method for triaging inpatients is key to a successful evacuation. A rational movement of patients from the inpatient unit to a staging area prior to transfer to another location/health care facility is necessary to move patients quickly and safely. It is essential, however, to realize that the triage priorities to which most clinical staff are accustomed in emergency response, i.e., the traditional START system, must be approached differently in an evacuation. Inpatients that are ambulatory and relatively stable will have first priority for moving off the inpatient nursing unit. These patients are less resource intensive, and many can be led off the unit with one or two staff members. Patients who are non-ambulatory, acutely ill, are unstable or require lifesaving equipment will require the most resources for moving.

As stated, for the purposed of evacuation triaging, the categories of START are reversed for the evacuation, however, they will revert to the original priority once the patient reaches the staging area prior to transfer, because you will want to get the most unstable patients moved to a health care facility first. An important consideration to take into account is how you get your medical equipment back. See the following chart for the prioritization:

Triage Level Chart

Triage Level	Priority for Evacuation off nursing unit: REVERSED START PRIORITY	Priority for Transfer to another healthcare facility: TRADITIONAL START PRIORITY
RED – STOP	These patience require maximum assistance to move. In an evacuation, these patients most LAST from the inpatient unit. These patients may require 2-3 staff members to transport	These patients require maximum support to sustain life in an evacuation. These patients move FIRST as transfers from your facility to another healthcare facility.
YELLOW – CAUTION	These patients require some assistance and should be moved SECOND in priority from the inpatient unit. Patients may require wheelchairs or stretchers and 1-2 staff members to transport	These patiens will be moved SECOND in priority as transfers from your facility to another health facility.
GREEN – GO	These patients require minimal assistance and can be moved FIRST from the unit. Patients are ambulatory and 1 staff member can safely lead several patients who fall into this category to the staging area.	These patients will be moved LAST as transfers from your facility to another healthcare facility.

These assessments must be made with clinical staff on the units. As the assessments are completed, it is recommended that the staff utilize a tagging system to clearly indicate what level of priority the patient has been given. Fluorescent tags, which are pre-strung, are one method of flagging patients. These can be affixed to the patient in some manner, one method being to apply these tags to the patient wrists (on the same arm as their patient ID band). The use of NCR paper with three copies should be considered in developing these tags, as this will assist in the reconciliation process. The tags can be imprinted with the patient's information using the patient's addressograph plate or labels with bar codes, depending on the system utilized in the organization, and as the patient moves from point to point, one of the copies can be torn off and used in the tracking and reconciliation process.

Tracking Tools

Tracking the movement of patients, staff, visitors and vendors throughout the organization during an evacuation is imperative to the reconciliation process that must occur to ensure that everyone has gotten out safely. Three tools were developed for this purpose:

‣ Patient Tracking tool

‣ Visitor Tracking tool

‣ Staff Tracking tool

The patient tracking tool should categorize the patients by location and indicate the level of care required during evacuation. Many states are now using electronic patient tracking tools.

The "Patient Care Unit Tracking Tool 1" documents the exact location of every patient ASSIGNED to the unit. This tool takes into account patients who may be off the floor at diagnostic tests or procedures, as well as patients who may still be in the emergency department or the Admitting office awaiting transport to the unit. This tool assists in the reconciliation of total patient census (assigned census) vs. actual census (patients present on the floor). The determination of whether a patient who is in the procedure area returns to the unit for evacuation or is evacuated from the procedure area to the staging area will be determined by the Incident Commander in consultation with the Unit Evacuation Leaders of each area.

"The Patient Care Unit Tracking Tool 2" documents the evacuation triage level assigned to the patient, as well as equipment needs, mode of transport, time of departure from the inpatient unit and time of arrival to the staging area.

The data should be sent electronically to the EOC, or mailed or brought to the attention of the Incident Commander, as well as to the staging area, to assist in reconciliation. In addition, the responsibility for tracking and reconciliation of patients will fall under the direction of the Patient Tracking Officer. Faxing could still be used, but as a redundant form of communication if Web-based tools are not available.

Tracking patient visitors, as well as others, who might be on the floor is equally important. Accounting for the staff also should be done in a methodical manner.

Designating When a Floor is Empty

It is important to validate that all patients and staff have been cleared from the patient unit, and then secure the floor.

The Unit Evacuation Leader should conduct a walk through of each room including support space. As each room is checked, it is recommended that some method of indicating that the room is empty is utilized. This can easily be accomplished by affixing a sticker or posting a sign (perhaps a large "X") on each of the doors within the area.

Identifying and Readying Patients for Evacuation from the Inpatient Unit

Medical Information

The transfer of critical patient information from one geographic area to another, as well as to other health care facilities, is important. In such a scenario, there will not be time for providers to review patient medical records or even transfer these records with the patient. Therefore, a summary of the pertinent information is required. Health care organizations that utilize electronic medical records should consider including an emergency patient summary in their planning and installation of such systems. However, it should also be recognized that, in the event an evacuation is necessary, electronic systems may be down, so extracting this information will become impossible and, therefore, manual methods must be identified.

The brief summary should be completed prior to moving the patient, and copies of critical pieces of information should go with it including:

‣ Copy of Medication Administration Sheets

‣ Copy of most recent set of complete medical orders

‣ Copies of latest lab reports

‣ Copy of DNR

‣ Copy of Advanced Directives

‣ Restraint Orders

‣ Baker Act documents

Medical Records

> The hospital must ensure that a process is in place to secure medical records.

This should be discussed with the Medical Records department, and policies should be developed that address the securing and transfer of records. There are three areas that should be addressed in formulating a policy to deal with the securing of medical records:

‣ **Old/Discharged Records:** Distinction needs to be made between active records and inactive records (patients who have previously been discharged but whose records have not been forwarded to Medical Records). Medical Record personnel should work with unit staff to collect all medical records on the unit. These records should be placed in a storage box and appropriately marked with a permanent marker.

‣ **Active patients Medical Records:** As patients are readying to leave the patient care unit, the

  ▷ Medical Record staff should collect all active medical records on the unit. These should be placed in a storage box and appropriately marked with a permanent marker. (Active Medical Records - Name of Patient Care Unit).

‣ **Split Medical Records:** Consideration needs to be given to split charts. Split Charts are medical record documents that are part of the patient's current hospitalization but, due to volume (most usually from prolonged hospitalization), non-urgent information has been removed from the active chart and stored elsewhere. The Medical Records staff must work with the unit staff to collect all split medical records on the unit. These should also be placed in a storage box and appropriately marked with a permanent marker. (Split Medical Records - Name of Patient Care Unit).

It is also recommended that once secured, the medical records be safeguarded from water damage. Boxes of medical records can be placed in clear plastic bags which are then sealed in order to protect them from water damage. Clear plastic bags should be utilized so that the markings on the boxes can be easily viewed.

Medications

It should be recognized that several hours may elapse until transportation to another health care organization is accomplished, and provisions for critical medications to be made available at the staging area is essential.

 Must Do ━━━━━━━━━━━━━

Hospitals must work with their pharmacies to identify what medications need to accompany patients and/or be available in the patient staging area.

In addition, emergency medications and equipment to address cardiac and respiratory arrests must also be provided at the staging area. It is recommended that, in drafting these policies, hospitals work with their pharmacies to ensure the movement of critical lifesaving medications and equipment.

Finally, the transferring facility should assess if the receiving facility has specific patient medications. In the instance where a specific patient medication is critical and not available at the receiving institution, the sending facility's pharmacy department should arrange to transfer the medication to the receiving facility.

Evacuation Toolkits

Pulling together the materials, documents and supplies to assist in evacuating a patient care floor cannot be left to the last minute. Each health care organization should consider assembling an evacuation toolkit for each patient care area and keeping this with their emergency equipment, for example with their Code carts.

Support Services Issues

Comprehensive evacuations plans should give consideration to the following areas and ensure that plans are in place to address each:

▸ **Systematic shutdown of medical gases, utilities and generators:** plans must include the procedures for shutting down and securing gases, electricity and water, not only floor by floor as they become evacuated, but entire buildings as they empty.

▸ **Telecommunication systems for relocated areas:** As units evacuate to staging areas, it is critical that alternate forms of communications be utilized. Publication of staging area phone numbers in the plan is one method. Hospitals can also consider using their redundant communication plans, as well (i.e., two way radios and/or cell phones).

▸ **Supplies:** Plans should be drafted that ensure that medical supplies, food, water and linen are moved to the staging area for patients.

▸ **Security:** finally plans should address the securing of floors, buildings and equipment to protect the assets of the hospital.

Writing an Emergency Plan

The Plan Outline

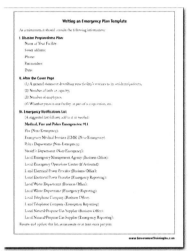

Staff Evacuation Template

Blank Forms are available online. Please see Table of Contents for instructions.

Building Directory Inventory for Evacuation Template

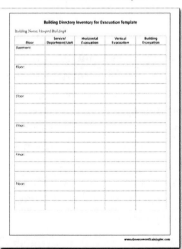

Departmental Evacuation Template

Patient Care Unit Evacuation Template   **Visitor Tracking Evacuation Template**

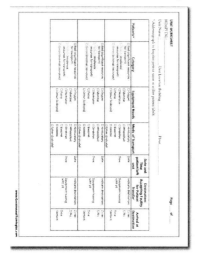

Blank Forms are available online. Please see Table of Contents for instructions.

General Evacuation Guidelines

During an emergency, initial evacuation of persons in immediate danger must take precedence over all other actions. Initial evacuation routes should be posted at the hospital's Nursing stations. Initiation of a vertical or complete evacuation of the hospital, with the exception of the need to move persons in immediate danger, should be coordinated under the direction of the hospital's Incident Commander. Incident specific evacuation routes and the process by which floors should be evacuated must be coordinated through a hospital's Incident Commander.

 Remember ─────────────

During a major emergency, a hospital's telephone service may be overloaded or disrupted. In such an event, the person responsible for hospital communications should ensure consistent communication.

The Communications Department should handle and coordinate internal communications and serve as a focal point for incoming and outgoing calls. In addition, the Communications Department, with the support of Security, should provide emergency communications equipment, such as radio systems, public address systems and portable radio units, for communications between employees throughout the emergency and for contacting emergency personnel. Evacuation and specific guidance for travel route and in-house transportation must be a systematic, coordinated effort in order to remove all patients, visitors and staff from the facility in a safe and timely manner.

A hospital should assign a designated, trained representative to the affected department(s) or unit discharge/exit point. This individual should be able to help provide in-house transportation information and real-time guidance required to move patients to the appropriate Refuge or Triage Areas within the facility. This individual should maintain radio contact with the assigned representative within the facility (e.g., Emergency Operations Center (EOC) via Logistics Chief) and relay information regarding departmental conditions and needs. They will maintain contact with the EOC throughout the incident or until evacuation of the area is complete.

Note: Communication with the Command Center is necessary at all times.

Evacuation Responsibilities

The Incident Commander or representative assigned for an incident should retain the full authority and remain responsible for the decision-making process until relieved by a more senior ranking official. Evacuation responsibilities for specific departments are summarized next.

All Hospital Employees

If a disaster occurs in a patient care area, or threatens a patient care area, employees should remove patients who are in immediate danger. DO NOT WAIT FOR INSTRUCTIONS. Patients should be taken to the nearest safe area on the same floor, if possible (horizontal evacuation). If the patients are not in immediate danger and the alarm has been activated, WAIT for evacuation orders.

Do not leave patients unattended. It should be ensured that hospital staff members assume responsibility for patients under someone else's care before they leave to report to pre-assigned disaster response assignments. For example, appropriate hand-off must be conducted before leaving any patient.

Security Department

All members of a hospital's Security Department should immediately communicate with their department for a head count and to receive emergency orders. Communication should be done by radio or telephone. They should be prepared to perform a variety of duties, including but not limited to:

- Ensure that an officer is dispatched to the designated area to meet the emergency responders and direct them to the scene of the problem. The main entrance is not a good location.
- Ensure that officers are dispatched as needed to direct entrances/exits and activate lock-down procedures for the facility, as written in the plan.
- Security officers should follow their Security Emergency Operations Procedures Manual.
- Security staff, using radios or an alternate communications system, should be located at exit(s) of patient care units to ensure that all patients, visitors and staff are accounted for, as per the plan.

Labor Pool

A representative should contact the facility's Emergency Operations Center (EOC). Normal visiting hours will be suspended during the disaster situation. It is anticipated that a significant number of people will volunteer their help during an emergency, including family members, visitors and nearby residents. The Human Services department or Planning Officer at the facility should help manage this influx and assign personnel to register these volunteers and assign them to a specific Staging Area. They should be prepared to perform a variety of duties, including but not limited to:

▸ Report to the Planning Officer or other representative assigned at the hospital for a head count and to receive emergency assignments.

▸ Manage and establish the control centers and staging areas for volunteers, patient families/visitors and medical students.

▸ Record volunteers' level of fitness, as they may be needed to transport patients up and down stairs.

▸ Ensure that responsible personnel are assigned to stay with relatives of victims in the hospital waiting area, and provide the EOC with the names of family members and volunteers that are in the facility.

▸ All volunteers should sign-in at the facility and should provide their full name, contact information, credentials and list any special talents - especially knowledge of another language.

Building Services

Building Services or other maintenance personnel should report to the leadership of their assigned work unit. They should be prepared to perform a variety of duties, including but not limited to:

▸ Help move patients, and assist as directed by the unit leadership.

▸ Maintain staffing of elevators and coordinate support from Security, as needed.

▸ Ensure that hallways or traffic areas are clear of carts and equipment and be responsible for setting up extra beds, if needed.

▸ Transport storeroom supplies and bring in resources from other areas of the facility, as requested.

▸ In the event of a facility-wide evacuation, the representative should be expected to help move patients and victims from patient rooms to refuge/treatment areas, and then to ambulances or other vehicles, as appropriate. Canvass organization for existing patient transport equipment and redirect, as needed, to critical areas. Ensure adequate number of stretchers and other equipment to move patients.

▸ Perform other duties as requested or redeploy to provide labor resources, as needed.

Food Services

Food Service employees at the facility should be prepared to perform a variety of duties, including but not limited to:

▸ Assist in directing visitors in the food service areas to exit the hospital.

▸ Immediately clear hallways of all tray carts, steam carts and food serving carts.

▸ Prepare and serve nourishment to patients, family members, volunteers and other personnel, if good health practices can be maintained.

▸ Set up menus or backup service in disaster situation and maintain adequate supplies.

▸ Evaluate the impact of the disaster situation to determine if utilities and appliances in kitchen and cafeteria areas should be shut off and are safe.

Facilities Management

The Facility Department or other assigned department representative at the facility should be prepared to perform a variety of duties, including but not limited to:

▸ Stand by to ensure shutdown of gas valves, heating, ventilation, air conditioning and other facility equipment, as appropriate.

▸ Maintain and control functioning of all available elevators, ventilation equipment and emergency generators.

▸ Be available to set up extra beds in hospital, if needed.

▸ Assume additional duties, as needed.

Facility Evacuation

Evacuation Of Non-Patient Areas

Should an incident occur of such magnitude requiring total evacuation from the building, or evacuation of a specific floor, the staff personnel on that floor should immediately evacuate to a safe area at the facility such as an Assembly/Staging Area, to await specific emergency response assignments. For purposes of identification, staff members of these non-patient care areas should be classified as non-clinical. Under emergency conditions, this group of personnel should report to the designated Staging Area (as determined by the hospital's Incident Commander) to receive emergency response assignments if they do not have pre-designated duties. General facility evacuation guidelines should include:

▸ Persons in immediate danger should vacate first via the nearest exit. Prior to opening an interior door, first using the back of your hand, feel the door for heat. NEVER open a door that feels hot to the touch. Try to find an alternative exit. Pull the fire alarm if you see fire, smoke or any hazardous condition.

▸ In threatened areas, first close all windows and doors if you can do so without placing yourself in danger.

▸ In an area where there are visitors, calmly gather them in one area and direct them in a single file to the nearest exit. Assign one volunteer or employee to lead them, and one volunteer or employee to be the last in line. These visitors should be sent or escorted to one of the pre-designated Assembly Areas in the facility. Visitors should remain in the assembly area until an "all clear" communication is declared or other directions are given. Available staff should then report their availability to the assigned Staging Area.

▸ Always close doors you pass through.

- Once you have reached a safe area of refuge, a call should be placed to the operator and the exact location of the hazard area should be given.

- Make provisions in the plan for vendors, students, contractors and others. What is their role? How should they respond?

Evacuating Patient Care Areas

During an evacuation of patient areas, patients should be prioritized for evacuation in the following manner:

1. Patients in Immediate Danger

2. Ambulatory Patients

3. Wheelchairs, Isolettes and Cribs

4. Bed Bound Patients

Response to a disaster situation should typically be addressed by one or more of the following:

Shelter in Place: Based upon the type of building construction and fire protection systems in the facility, staff, patients and visitors may be instructed to remain where they are until further instructions are provided to them. Closing doors and windows in patient rooms should provide initial protection from fire. In most incidents, the safest place for a patient is in his/her room.

> NEVER hesitate to relocate because of imminent danger.

Certain instructions may be given to maintain order and keep everyone informed of the latest status of the incident. Initiation of the Shelter-in-Place policy requires that all routine activities stop and that preparations are made to enable immediate movement of patients should the incident necessitate such actions, as outlined in the following types of patient evacuation.

Horizontal Evacuation (sometimes called relocation): This stage involves patients who are secured from immediate danger but remain on the same floor. Horizontal evacuation typically means that everyone in the Unit should be moved to the opposite side of the building.

Vertical Evacuation: This stage refers to the complete evacuation of a floor. For a localized incident, occupants can be transferred to an area of refuge identified elsewhere in the hospital, typically at least two floors beneath the incident floor. In the case of a complete facility evacuation, occupants should be removed to the assigned Refuge Area. All patients should be tagged and/or triaged by designated leadership before they leave their floor.

Total Evacuation: This stage involves the complete evacuation of the facility. Total evacuation should be initiated only as a last resort. Patients should be transferred to alternate locations and facilities. This decision should require coordination between all sections operating under the facility's Hospital Emergency Incident Command System (HEICS).

Evacuation Levels

Any employee, who reasonably believes that an emergency is taking place, or is about to take place, that could put patients or staff in imminent danger, should initiate the emergency evacuation of an area. When the fire alarm sounds, employees should be expected to implement the fire response protocol appropriate to his or her work area. There is no code to indicate if an alarm signifies a drill or real fire. Therefore, every alarm should be treated as a potentially serious event.

Clinical Department Requirements

General Standards

▸ Maintain continuity of care by assigning responsibilities for ancillary personnel assigned to the unit which may include: Transport, Housekeeping and Laundry, Respiratory, Food/Nutrition, Materials Management, Central Services, etc., and request additional resources, as needed.

▸ Report to or assign staff to communicate with the Emergency Operations Center (EOC).

▸ Request additional personnel to support and transport patients, especially during nights and weekend shifts.

▸ Provide adequate drug and medical equipment (e.g., Propaq, oxygen, IV pump, etc.) to support each patient during transportation and evacuation procedures.

▸ Assign staff to clear all obstructions from corridors, and then stand by to control fire/smoke doors and exits, as required.

▸ Coordinate the discharge and movement of current patients to create room for incoming patients or evacuees from other areas in the hospital.

▸ Evacuate patients in immediate danger first, including OB, followed by ambulatory patients. Appoint a helper to go with them and lead them to the safest part of the same floor (toward exit). Direct the leader as to where to take the patients if they must leave the floor. Do not leave ambulatory patients without staff guidance. When possible, use wheelchairs to remove non-ambulatory patients to a safe place on the same level, and then take the chairs back for additional patients. Plan for patients in restraints, forensic patients and so on.

▸ The immediate safety of the patient at this time must be given preference over aseptic techniques.

▸ As unit is evacuated, assess the need to shut off utilities (e.g., medical gases, equipment, lighting, etc.).

▸ Be alert for further instructions or changing environment hazards. Make periodic checks to assess patients' safety and emotional health.

▸ Ensure that doors are closed and mark an "X" (with a grease pencil or tape) after a patient room is evacuated. Your hospital may have other ways of annotating that a room has been evacuated – but most nurses have access to tape.

▸ Before initiating a horizontal evacuation of patients, supervisors should do a quick check of the adjoining area of refuge to avoid unnecessary movement to potentially unsafe areas.

▸ In collaboration with physicians, evaluate the condition of each patient.

▸ Secure a triage transportation tag to the patient gown or robe; provide a copy of the tag to Patient Access for tracking (not applicable in a horizontal evacuation, as staff should accompany patients).

▸ Determine the best available method for transportation for each patient and most appropriate destination based on patient acuity and care needs (e.g., SNF, etc).

▸ Identify and procure specialty equipment that will be necessary for transportation and continued patient care, as needed.

▸ If time, place patient records, medications, clothing and valuables in a bag with each patient's name clearly marked in indelible ink on the bag. Otherwise, just go!

▸ Assist Patient Access and Social Services in notifying patient emergency contact.

If horizontal evacuation is implemented, it could be just the initial step in a series of movements to safety. Be alert for further instructions!

Medical and Surgical Patient Care Units

Staff on general and specialty care units need to anticipate rapid disconnection of equipment. This will include what is critical to transport, what can be left behind and how to safely "package" the patient with their equipment for transport.

Requirements for Evacuation: When an emergency occurs, nursing staff members at the facility should report to their own department for a head count and emergency assignments. The Unit Nurse Manager or designated leadership responsible for nursing staff in a particular unit should direct activities of the Unit staff. These activities may include, but are not limited to:

Unit Specific Standards

Orthopedic patients who are fastened into traction devices may not fit through doorways. To the extent possible, patients should not be left unattended. Ropes and straps may have to be cut to move the patient.

Operating Rooms, Post Anesthesia Care Units and Hemodialysis

The following personnel are responsible for ensuring the safety of all patients:

▸ Operating suite, the surgeon in charge in each case.

▸ PACU, the covering anesthesiologist is responsible to coordinate with nursing.

▸ Hemodialysis unit, Nursing is responsible.

The Unit Nurse Manager or designated leadership will direct activities of the Unit staff. These activities may include, but are not limited to:

Unit Specific Standards

▸ Close doors to occupied OR suite(s), and place wet towels around the doors if smoke, dust or fumes are present; keep the surgeon advised on safe exit routes, relocation or refuge areas.

▸ To the greatest extent possible, obtain equipment and services required for completion of the surgery; keep a list of anticipated supplies on hand and be prepared to ensure additional sterile supplies can be processed quickly.

OR/PACU Nights and Weekend Shift/Hemodialysis Unit:

▸ Immediately call for additional support to transport and move patients.

▸ Evacuate ambulatory patients first. Gather these patients together and have them form a chain by holding hands.

▸ Appoint a helper to go with ambulatory patients and lead them to the safest part of the same floor (toward exit). Direct the leader where to take them if they must leave the floor.

▸ Do not leave ambulatory patients without staff guidance. When possible, use wheelchairs to remove non-ambulatory patients to a safe place on the same level conference room, and then return the chairs for remaining patients. Non-ambulatory patients may be rolled in a blanket and moved to a safe location.

Intensive Care Units

Requirements for Evacuation:

In the event of an emergency, the Unit Nurse Manager or designated leadership must evaluate patients in the Intensive Care Units in collaboration with intensivist or medical/surgical house staff for possible discharge. Using established discharge criteria as a guide, as many patients as possible should be transferred out of the Intensive Care Units. The Unit Nurse Manager or designated leadership should direct activities of the Unit staff. These activities may include, but are not limited to:

Unit Specific Standards

▸ Patients may be rolled in a blanket and dragged to a safe location in addition to using stretchers and beds where feasible;

▸ Work with medical/surgical house staff and respiratory therapists to evaluate whether it is appropriate to shut-off oxygen, ventilation equipment and other gases and provide interim support.

▸ Children should be handled like other patients, except that in ambulatory evacuation alternate the older and younger children in the evacuation line, if time and circumstances permit.

Labor and Delivery Units

Requirements for Evacuation:

Designated Nursing staff members should report to their own department for a head count and emergency assignments. The Unit Nurse Manager or designated leadership will direct activities of the Unit staff. These activities may include, but are not limited to:

Unit Specific Standards

▸ Assign support staff to wheel incubators, instruments and supplies with the patient, if needed, to complete Labor and Delivery procedures.

▸ Many hospitals now have a system where you can place eight bassinets on a stretcher – two babies per bassinet – accompanied by two nurses. Provisions have to be made for mothers after C-sections who may still have an epidural catheter in place.

Mother-Baby Unit, Pediatrics, NICU AND PICU

Requirements for Evacuation:

In the event of an emergency, the Unit Nurse Manager or designated leadership should ensure that as many babies as possible are taken to their mothers. The Unit Nurse Manager or designated leadership should direct activities of the Unit staff. These activities may include, but are not limited to:

Unit Specific Standards

▸ Boarder babies will remain in cribs/bassinets with a nurse in attendance during defend in place and horizontal evacuations.

▸ Incubator babies should be moved in their incubators to other locations, and, if necessary, multiple babies may be placed into a single crib or incubator.

Evacuation Transportation Tag

An Evacuation Transportation Tag System can be useful to track patients who require evacuation from the facility. Physicians and Nursing staff at your facility should be responsible for patient assessment/triage which will dictate mode of transportation based on acuity and care needs.

Conditions permitting, the assessment/triage process and transportation tag completion should be completed prior to movement of patients from hospital. The tags should be updated and referred to during triage and transportation to the areas of refuge and possibly other health care facilities.

Patient Access or designated representative at the facility should be responsible for:

▸ Maintaining a supply of the evacuation tags.

▸ Coordinating the distribution of evacuation tags during an event.

▸ Tracking patients who are being transported to other locations.

Transportation Resources

Transportation needs should be assessed, and appropriate types of vehicles (ambulance, ambulette, van, etc.) will be determined. The Transportation Officer or other assigned representative should coordinate travel arrangements through contracted vendors.

Transportation requirements for large numbers of patients, medical supplies and equipment are difficult. In addition, available relocation sites with the necessary advanced life support equipment and emergency medical facilities tend to be scarce. The contracts with transportation resources/services should be reviewed and renewed on a regular basis.

Additional transportation resources might be available via contact with the Office of Emergency Management). However, this will depend on the nature of the event and its effect on citywide/state resources.

The need for activation of EMS mutual aid agreements between one city and surrounding EMS agencies (even out of state), such as commercial and volunteer agencies, may be required to augment the EMS and transportation resources available to your facility and others during an event.

Alternate Care Sites

A list of hospital affiliations should be kept and made available during an event. The most prominent issue, as is the case with many hospitals, is that of staffing, specifically nurses, for the extra beds and even for existing beds.

The Centers for Bioterrorism Preparedness Planning (CBPP) affiliated hospitals in New York have a memorandum of agreement to serve as alternate care sites for each other if the need arises. Examples of such needs include but are not limited to: surge capacity, decontamination and special populations. Review all agreements.

For long-distance evacuation, consider air support. U.S. Air Ambulance, based in Sarasota, Florida, which focuses on finding the most appropriate mode of transportation – air ambulance, long-distance ground ambulance, commercial medical escorts by train and air and international stretcher service on commercial airlines. They have also established the Hospital Evacuation Liaison Program (HELP) for hospitals and nursing homes. The program addresses the logistical difficulties inherent in mass patient evacuation, including locating and contracting with patient transport providers and receiving hospitals. There are also organizations of amateur pilots able to assist in evacuations in emergencies.

📋 Checklist

Local Government (EOC) Evacuation Checklist

Situation Assessment

☐ Determine type, size and location of emergency.

☐ Determine number of people affected.

☐ Determine emergency assistance required, especially for vulnerable populations.

Infrastructure Assessment

☐ Conduct infrastructure assessment (public and high-risk buildings).

- o Transportation

- o Communications

- o Utilities

Evacuation

☐ Identify areas to be evacuated.

☐ Identify transportation/roadways to be used.

☐ Alert local law enforcement, Highway Patrol, and local and state transportation authorities.

☐ Identify vulnerable populations, including people from unique institutions to be evacuated.

Alert and Warning / Notification

☐ Determine if thresholds for alert and warning have been reached.

☐ Consider announcing precautionary warnings for vulnerable populations (hospitals, nursing homes/care facilities, schools, special event facilities, etc.).

☐ Identify whether the emergency affects life and property.

☐ Activate public warning system: Emergency Alert System, including emergency digital information system (EDIS).

☐ Issue public advisory notification.

☐ Advise Operational Area (city/county) of situation.

☐ Advise affected jurisdictions, agencies and facilities of public evacuation.

Initial Response

☐ Announce a precautionary warning for vulnerable populations.

☐ Declare a local emergency.

☐ Issue local emergency orders/evacuation order.

☐ Close affected areas.

Public Information

☐ Issue precautionary warnings and instructions for vulnerable populations.

☐ Issue evacuation instructions.

☐ Issue news releases.

☐ Issue press advisories.

Mass Care and Shelter

Identify sheltering needs and capabilities.

☐ Activate/establish multi-jurisdictional agreements for care and shelter.

☐ Activate existing agreements with American Red Cross, Salvation Army and community-based organizations.

☐ designate shelter areas:

  o Medical treatment unit/temporary infirmary, and

  o General public shelters.

Partial

Dependent upon the location, extent and type of emergency, a partial evacuation may be ordered by Emergency Management on the scene. Only those persons located in the immediate vicinity of the emergency will be moved to a location out of the area of possible danger, as follows:

▸ Patients and staff are to be evacuated beyond the nearest set of fire doors.

▸ Floors above and below the immediate area may be evacuated, if necessary.

▸ If the affected area is a patient care floor, the Unit Director, Charge Nurse or Director shall:

  ▷ Designate one employee to salvage medical records.

  ▷ Designate one employee to ensure all patients and staff are evacuated and accounted for, using patient census report or appointment schedules.

  ▷ Ensure that all patients are assigned a caregiver to monitor condition and provide care, as needed.

▸ If the affected area is an office, lab or any other general service, the Manager, Director or Supervisor shall ensure that all employees are evacuated and accounted for.

▸ All windows and doors should be closed when leaving the evacuated area.

Complete

In the event that the facility has suffered structural damage or is in imminent danger of this, is unable to provide basic utilities needed to sustain services, or a circumstance should render the building as unsafe, a complete evacuation may be ordered. The following guidelines are designed to be flexible as circumstances may dictate:

Communication

An appropriate public address announcement shall be ordered by Emergency Management.

Patient Evaluation

Nursing and House Staff shall evaluate patients for immediate discharge to reduce the number of patients to be transported.

Evacuation Procedures

On patient care floors, the Unit Director, Charge Nurse or Director shall designate employees to salvage any hard copies of medical records and employees to ensure all patients and staff are evacuated and accounted for, using patient census report or appointment schedules. This may be necessary if the EMR system is down.

In an office, lab or any other general service, the Manager, Director or Supervisor shall ensure that all employees are evacuated and accounted for and vital records are removed. In anesthetizing and surgical areas, the surgeon, in cooperation with Emergency Management must decide to either terminate or proceed with surgeries. If surgery is terminated, disconnect the monitoring and support systems. The head nurse will designate a team of loaders and movers to relocate patients to evacuation staging areas, following departmental policies for evacuation of patients. All other patient care areas should refer to their departmental policies for the evacuation of patients. All windows and doors should be closed when leaving the area.

Staging Area

Depending on the area affected, all Hospital areas will evacuate to the Clinic on the same floor; all Clinic areas will evacuate to the Hospital on the same floor. The Director or Supervisor of each receiving floor shall supervise the receiving of patients and staff. The staging areas are temporary, to be used until transportation is arranged for patients to be transported to a designated alternate care site, or for non-admit patients and visitors to provide their own transportation. Staging areas are not intended as overnight or long-term treatment areas. If the Hospital or Clinic does not require immediate evacuation, patients will remain until transportation is ready.

Admissions Department shall maintain a disposition log of each patient (i.e., transported to what facility, discharged home, etc.).

Utilities and Supply Management

Facilities Management shall provide minimal electrical hookups for equipment such as pumps, ventilators, monitors, etc. Facilities Management shall be prepared to shut off and reactivate building utilities. Gas and ventilation may be shut off for fire prevention.

‣ Respiratory Therapy shall provide portable oxygen, as needed.

‣ Laundry and Environmental Services shall provide linen and beds, as needed.

‣ Basic medical supplies will be furnished by Central Supply, Nursing and Pharmacy.

‣ Elevator Use

Visitor and service elevators shall be used to evacuate semi-ambulatory and non-ambulatory patients ONLY. Ambulatory patients shall use stairwells to descend to ground floor or other, if necessary. Usually there are limited elevators on emergency power.

Transportation

Transportation of ambulatory patients and accompanying staff shall be available through Transportation Services and internal shuttle busses. Transportation of non-ambulatory patients and accompanying staff shall be arranged in liaison with local authorities, ambulance services and so on.

If additional resources are needed, the DHH Office of Public Health EMS line should be contacted for assistance.

The charge nurse will assign a caregiver to accompany each patient during evacuation and transportation.

Security

Evacuees or unauthorized personnel shall not be allowed to re-enter any evacuated area. If after the emergency has ended, the building is deemed not safe for occupancy, Security shall be responsible for preventing unauthorized personnel from entering.

Alternate Care Site

If evacuation of the facility becomes necessary, the Incident Command Center will facilitate evacuation to another facility.

Patient transportation, tracking and management of patient records shall be the responsibility of the transferring facility until patients are received at the alternate care facility.

The Medical Director will determine the order in which patients are evacuated from the hospital. Ideally, depending on availability of transport, equipment and personnel, etc., the order should be mothers and newborns, ICU, Dialysis, Surgical, Medical, Psychiatry, DNR and Hospice/terminally ill.

The Medical Director, Chief Operations Officer or other ICC member shall inform the alternate care facility that an evacuation is under way, the approximate number of patients that will be transported and the estimated time of the first arrivals.

Admissions Department shall keep a master list of final patient disposition of all evacuated patients.

Operating Room Evacuation Procedures

In anesthetizing and surgical areas, the surgeon, in cooperation with the Hospital Command Center Medical Specialist (such as the Chief of Medical Staff), must decide to either terminate or proceed with the procedure.

Neighborhood Clinic and Other Off-Campus Location Evacuation

These locations shall follow guidelines in Partial Evacuation and Complete Evacuation with exceptions as follows:

▸ Manager/Director of location is authorized to order evacuation and initiate action, in place of the Emergency Management.

▸ All evacuees shall be assembled in a pre-designated location.

Members	Responsibilities
Anesthesia Board Runner	Assign additional personnel at the scene as needed (in conjunction with Charge Nurse).
Anesthesiologist/CRNA	Gather necessary supplies and drugs from anesthesia cart.
	Switch to portable tanks and order shut off of wall supply.
	Responsible for patient during the move; maintain respiration of patient during the move
Charge Nurse	Designate a team of loaders and movers to relocate to evacuation areas, following departmental policies for evacuation of patients.
	Assign additional personnel, as needed.
Hospital Command Center	Determine, with Surgeon, to either terminate or proceed with the procedure. Communicate with OR Desk to appraise fire situation (if evacuation is due to a fire).

Members	Responsibilities
Operating Room Assistant/Anesthesia Tech	Assist with physical movement of equipment, i.e., OR table, anesthesia machine, as designated by circulator.
	Assist anesthesiologist on high-risk cases, i.e., CV-Craniotomies, total joints or major spinal cases with equipment to be transported.
	Disconnect monitors.
	Disconnect IVs from poles.
	Obtain transport monitors, where necessary.
	Obtain equipment to be needed in destination.
Resident/Assisting Surgeon	Responsible for movement of table or stretcher.
	Responsible for safety of the patient.
RN Circulator	Activate alarm if in his/her area.
	Help with disconnecting the anesthesia machine in preparation for evacuation.
	Assist with transporting anesthesia machine if no anesthesia tech available.
Scrub Nurse\Surgical Tech	Gather necessary surgical instruments and equipment from mayo stand and back table, place on patient.
	Assist in moving operating table or stretcher.
Surgeon	Will decide with Hospital Command Center either to terminate or proceed with surgeries.
	Stabilize operative site.
	Give final order to move.
	Determine if medical gasses need to be culled at the zone valve.

Communications

It is essential to have plans in place for reliable communications between key personnel during any emergency.

It is also important to have an efficient information network in place to keep all stakeholders informed, especially staff, patients and their families, and the media.

Information Centers can establish a Website to keep people informed. Maximum use should be made of social media to get key messages out and keep people informed. You can set up an information center within the facility to provide the latest information about the emergency.

It is also essential to keep the media informed, although this must be coordinated by the emergency team and handled according to your crisis communications plan. Only designated spokespersons should speak with the media, and only agreed statements should be released.

Simplicity, credibility, verifiability, consistency and speed count when communicating in the initial phases of the crisis. The initial phase of a crisis is characterized by confusion and intense media interest. Information is usually incomplete and the facts are dispersed. It is important to recognize that information from the media, other organizations and within your organization may not be accurate. Your role is to learn the facts about what happened, to determine your organization's response to the problem and to verify the true magnitude of the event as quickly as possible. In the initial phase, there is no second chance to get it right. Your organization's reputation depends on what you do and do not say, and on when or whether you say it.

As the crisis evolves, anticipate sustained media interest and scrutiny. Unexpected developments, rumors, or misinformation may place further media demands on organization communicators. Experts, professionals and others not associated with your organization will comment publicly on the issue and sometimes contradict or misinterpret your messages. Expect to be criticized about your handling of the situation. Staying on top of the information flow and maintaining tight coordination are essential. Processes for tracking communication activities become increasingly important as the workload increases.

Incident Log (or Command Center Log)

The log should contain relevant facts with dates and times and actions taken. A separate media log should be maintained in which all media calls are logged. These entries should contain the name of the journalist, time of the call, the questions asked and responses given. All team members should contribute to both logs, so that the most detailed record is kept.

 Remember ─────────────

It is important to keep a detailed log as the crisis develops.

By reviewing the media log you can determine from the questions how the media are approaching the crisis. Then, by analyzing their articles and news reports, you can see how they are responding to your answers. Reviewing the logs will also tell you which journalists are covering the crisis. You may have a better relationship with some than with others. The editorials will also provide insight into how a particular news media views the crisis. If the article or editorial is unfair or inaccurate, you must try to speak to the person involved in order to set the record straight. Always try to contact the journalist first, and, if that isn't successful, speak to the editor.

FEMA has an ICS form (214) log that can be used to document activities and their timeframe.

Critical Incident Stress Management

Critical Incident Stress Management is a comprehensive, systematic and multi-component approach to managing traumatic stress within an organization. It is designed to maintain and enhance the health of an organization's personnel and is an essential part of the good management of any organization.

In the event of a disaster/emergency event requiring incident stress debriefing, specially trained peer support personnel, under the direction of the Psychological Support Unit Leader, will provide support services for Health First associates patients, and families. When necessary, the local authority will assist with these services.

Evacuation To Alternate Care Site Procedure

Evacuation refers to the movement of patients and personnel from the hospital, or any of its components, in as rapid and safe a manner as possible under the existing situation for transfer of patients to an alternate care site – within the hospital is preferred. Reasons for evacuation include removing patients and personnel from actual or threatened danger and to free hospital beds/facilities for care of incoming casualties. Under most circumstances, there will not be a total evacuation of the hospital. Every effort will be made to move patients to another safer location within the hospital. Total evacuation will only be considered as a last resort.

Alternatives to Hospital Evacuations

▸ **Partial or localized evacuation:** When portions of a facility are determined unsafe by the Logistics Section Chief, the Hospital President will order evacuation of patients and staff to safe unaffected areas of the hospital.

▸ **Shelter in place:** This involves shutting windows and closing ventilation systems to outside airflows. A hazardous materials incident with airborne threat is a possible cause.

▸ **Assignment of additional resources to ensure safe levels of service:** A timely identification of required assistance due to loss of vital services, medical gases or damage to the facility. Allocation of governmental and/or private industry resources will alleviate the need for partial or complete evacuation.

▸ **Creation of safety buffer zone around the hospital:** Sufficient resources are positioned between the threat and the hospital to eliminate the need for evacuation or provide more time to effect a more safe and orderly evacuation. This is utilized during community emergency situations.

Categories of Evacuation

Immediate: Immediate public safety threat to the hospital requiring hospital closure and evacuation of patients and staff to temporary locations or other facilities, as quickly as possible, using all available resources. All alternatives to evacuation have been considered and are not acceptable to the Command Center Staff.

Priority: A major public safety threat to a hospital that will have a high probability of requiring hospital closure and evacuation of patients and staff to a temporary location or other facilities. Alternatives to evacuation are being executed to obtain more time to effect a safe and orderly evacuation. Priority evacuation orders originate with the Hospital President.

Extended: An extended evacuation process, possibly caused by degradation of utilities, damage to the hospital, or other causes. Time criteria will allow ambulance and other transportation resources to provide required transport of patients between temporary locations or other facilities and the hospital. The Hospital President will order and coordinate the procedure.

Authority and Responsibility for Evacuation

The Incident Commander(IC) or Administrator on Call is the person responsible for determining the need for hospital evacuation. The IC, if unavailable, may designate an alternate (this may be the administrator on call). This person, with vested authority as an Executive Officer can ensure that appropriate supplies, equipment and resources are mobilized and is in charge of Evacuation Operations.

The IC or the Administrator on Call is responsible for determining if evacuation will be necessary and for determining the scope of evacuation based on the escalation of the disaster or emergency situation. The IC will determine the time to notify the receiving hospitals based on current transfer agreements, urgency of the situation and status of beds within other group hospitals.

The amount of time required for evacuation to be completed depends entirely on the type of evacuation. In most situations only a portion of the hospital may have to be evacuated. The amount of time required to complete a partial evacuation is dependent upon the number of patients that have to be relocated. For planning purposes, it is estimated that a partial evacuation could be completed in 12 hours. In the event of a full hospital evacuation, a period of 48 hours should be allowed to complete the evacuation.

The 150-bed Cape Canaveral Hospital in Cocoa Beach, Florida, can do a complete evacuation in three to four hours and has had to many times as a planned hurricane event.

The IC or administrator on call is responsible for giving the order to evacuate patients based on their medical condition and stability in coordination with the Vice President of Medical Staff Affairs. The IC is responsible for ultimately closing the facility and for notifying executive members.

When the IC requires evacuation for whatever reason (hurricane, loss of water supply, loss of power supply or internal disaster), it will be coordinated with the County Director of Emergency Management and the Vice President of Medical Staff Affairs. Total evacuation is used only as a last resort. Physicians designated by the Vice President of Medical Staff Affairs will give designation of specific patients for evacuation.

Each Department Director is responsible for and will activate that particular department's plan for dealing with the disaster and evacuation, as indicated.

Types of Evacuation

▸ Evacuation by nursing units and floors:

▹ All patients in a nursing unit, regardless of condition, are moved from that unit to some other location(s) either within or outside the hospital. This type of evacuation might be required where there is an internal disaster or where there is an immediate threat of disaster to the whole hospital or any of its parts.

▹ Evacuation based on patient condition (ambulatory diagnostic problems, ambulatory observation cases, patients scheduled for discharge, etc.):

▹ Patients are removed from the hospital by stages, the least serious cases first, the next serious second, etc. This type of evacuation might be required to free beds and facilities for incoming casualties.

Priority System for Patient Evacuation:

▸ Several categories of patient evacuation must be considered for each emergency. These are:

▹ Patients that can be discharged immediately such as those admitted for elective surgery, pre-op or those near full recovery.

▹ Patients that can be evacuated by car, and/or bus in a sitting position.

▹ Patients that can be evacuated by van, bus or ambulance on stretchers or backboards.

▸ In cases where an internal disaster requires immediate evacuation of patients whose lives are endangered, patients may be moved to a safe area by the person discovering the emergency. The decision to move remaining patients on the nursing unit shall be made by the nurse in charge of the unit in conjunction with the physician (if present), charge nurse or unit manager.

▸ Determination of emergency power or electricity will be done to ensure that there is power to complete the evacuation. There are generators available that supply the hospital.

▸ Should natural gas be unavailable, a fuel supply is kept onsite for three days to feed the boilers. The kitchen does not have a backup of fuel, so in the absence of fuel or electricity, food would be served cold.

▸ If propane gas is used but unavailable, fuel oil is available, but would be shared with the generator. This would shorten the run time of the generator to four days and the boilers (one running) to four days. The kitchen does not have a backup of fuel, so in the absence of electricity, food would be served cold.

Evacuating to Another Hospital

In the event the hospital must be evacuated, the Hospital President (or designee) will advise as to location and routes. Examples are:

▸ To their homes (patients whose condition permits may be discharged).

▸ To another section of the hospital.

▸ To other hospitals.

▸ To nearby buildings.

▸ To reception points in other communities.

The IC or designee should first activate the disaster plan to prepare for evacuation. The Command Center will serve as the central location for all communication. Patients will be evaluated in the following manner in order to reduce the number of evacuees and/or to ensure available space for incoming hospital and emergency cases.

All patients that are capable of going home or are released to family/significant others are considered discharged. All other patients requiring additional medical support based on condition are considered transfers. Each clinical unit will fax a list of patients being discharged home and those requiring transfer to another facility to the Command Center. The Case Manager or Patient Advocate will notify family members as soon as absolutely possible regarding the plans for the patients.

Patients who require further care will be evaluated and moved to other hospitals under the direction of the Incident Commander, Operations Sections Chief and the Medical Staff Director.

The first consideration for an evacuation destination shall be another group hospital. This allows the patient to stay within the same patient tracking and status system. All records and documents will still be available electronically to appropriate personnel.

In the event of an evacuation to another facility, the Disaster Census Worksheet for Evacuation shall be used.

Communication is key between the departments. Should the online version of the worksheet be unavailable, a hard copy should be available from the Nursing Supervisors, and in the Disaster Manuals in each department. In this case, the units will fax or hand-carry the completed sheets to the appropriate locations.

Bed availability and staff will be verified before patients leave the hospital. All essential medical records and consent forms will be sent with the patient per policy. Nursing personnel (as appropriate), supplies, drugs and records, etc., will be transferred with these patients.

Receiving hospitals will be notified by the Command Center after the nursing units have called and given a report on the patient to double-check bed availability. The Liaison Officer will contact receiving facilities to inform of the approximate number of patients, estimated time of arrival, and will fax a patient list to the receiving facility.

The Operations Section Chief and the Medical Staff Director in coordination with the Director of Bed Control and the Supervisor of Admissions will maintain a master list of patients to be evacuated. Patients will be dispositioned on the nursing units and discharged through Bed Control. The Emergency Department will be one of the staging areas for patient evacuation to other facilities and will be the last area of the hospital to close.

The Hospital Command Center should initiate:

▸ Requests for medical staff office to work with physicians to obtain discharge or transfer orders. Case Management can assist with supporting discharge or transfer arrangements once the physicians have identified the disposition status for their patients.

▸ The Hospital Command Center Operations Chief can designate staff (including Case Management) to support notification of families of patients of their discharge or transfer status.

▸ Patient Transfer Checklist.

▸ Copy parts of Medical Records per the Patient Transfer to Other Facilities Policy in the Operations Manual. Medical Records personnel will be assigned to floors to assist with copying records and entering new information.

▸ Original chart to be sent to Medical Records Department.

▸ Obtain appropriate patient supplies, medications and IVs. Label and prepare to transport with patients.

▸ Evaluate surgery schedule for elective surgeries for the next 24 to 48 hours.

▸ Inventory departments to determine supplies needed, perishables to be reduced or discarded and storm preparations implemented to secure department.

Patient Staging Areas will be set up in the Emergency Department. These areas will be utilized in both patient evacuations and receiving patients after the disaster. Staging area personnel will have the following evacuation responsibilities:

▸ Staging Area Nurse - coordinates documents for patient transport.

▸ Floor nurse - completes patient transfer checklist.

▸ Medical Records - reviews transfer checklist for completeness.

▸ Patient Registrar - faxes face sheets and insurance cards to receiving facilities.

▸ Unit Secretary - notifies Command Center when patients are en route.

▸ Ambulance representatives - provides communication between Emergency Department, ambulances and receiving facilities.

A list of all patients requiring transfer to other facilities is to be forwarded to the Command Center. The list will include:

▸ Patients name and diagnosis

▸ Name and contact number of nearest relative

▸ Transportation method: ALS Ambulance, BLS Ambulance, Helicopter, hospital shuttle service, etc.

▸ Need for medical assistance during transport

▸ Patient preference for receiving facility (when appropriate)

▸ Name of attending physician

If necessary, hospital staff will accompany patients on transfers. This will be done based on patient condition and in accordance with hospital transfer policies. Patients requiring BLS and ALS support during transport will be released only to ambulance services with BLS/ALS state licensure.

In coordination with the Admitting Department, Medical Staff accompaniment of evacuated patients will be based on the medical condition of the patient on a case by case basis (in an ideal situation) and designated by the Vice President of Patient Care Services or designee.

In the event of a major evacuation of patients from the facility, every effort will be made to send with the patient a 72-hour supply of medications, as well as the patient's medical record. Food and water will not be transported to the receiving hospital unless specific agreements indicate otherwise.

All patients that are evacuated from the facility will have their armbands in place for identification purposes.

The Nurse Directors, Managers of the nursing unit and Security shall ensure all patients are evacuated and accounted for and (when the situation allows) secure each unit/department:

- Unplug all non-essential electrical equipment.
- Cover computers/monitors, and move any away from windows, if possible.
- Close all windows, blinds and doors.
- Inventory narcotics, and return to Pharmacy. Shut down Pyxis units.
- In the event of total evacuation, the following timeframe guidelines will be used:
- One hour prior to evacuation, notify vendors for additional equipment, resources and supplies (unless evacuation is immediate).
- Forty-eight-hour notices, depending on severity of the disaster and the amount of support and assistance received from outside agencies, for the hospital to complete evacuation.

Internal Disaster Evacuation

In case of an emergency evacuation of a nursing unit, all patients shall be moved immediately to another safe area of the hospital regardless of their condition. Ambulatory and semi-ambulatory patients shall be moved first, and then those that are bedridden.

Re-Entry to The Facility

The Incident Commander will be responsible for determining if the hospital can be reopened and to what level it will provide patient care. The IC, in coordination with the appropriate department directors and local county and state officials, will inspect the facility before reentry of patients and staff. This inspection will be conducted in consultation with AHCA.

Plans to reopen will be dependent on a number of factors, including access to the hospital, the amount of damage sustained by the building and equipment, the availability of personnel, and the availability of support systems, including electricity, water and communications.

Once access to the hospital has been restored, hospital administration will meet and tour the facility, determine damage and estimate time for repairs. Notification of associates, physicians and the general public will be made through media announcement. The Essential departments will be opened first. The hospital will cooperate with all agencies and relief agencies to facilitate recovery of the hospital as soon as safe.

Once the disaster or emergency situation is such that the hospital has been reopened, the master list of patients will be used to call the transferring facilities, and obtain condition information and assess for the possibility of return to the hospital.

 Remember ——————————————

This can be a slow process as some patients opt to stay at the receiving hospital rather than be transferred again and other patients may have been discharged. The command center does not have to be open for repatriation.

When a reopening time has been established, the Command Center will open. The Liaison Officer or designee will call the facilities that had received patients during the evacuation process to determine their current status. Patients remaining in those facilities will be given the option to stay at their current facility or to return. A priority list will be identified based on several factors including bed needs, staffing availability, and identified units to be reopened. Receiving hospitals will fax a list of all patients to return to the evacuating facility to the Command Center. The Operations Section Chief will maintain this list and coordinate assigning these patients to units/rooms. The Planning Section Chief will coordinate staffing of the Staging Areas for receiving patients and transport to the units. The Logistics Chief ensures coordination of patient transportation with transportation companies and arranges transportation devices (wheelchairs, gurneys, etc.) to be available to assist in reentry. The Security Officer will coordinate securing of areas for transport vehicles, coordinate traffic control and monitor entrances/exits for visitor/associate/patient control. The Medical Staff Director will confer with Operations Section Chief and Incident Commander, and coordinate with physicians the return of patients to their care.

Patients that require transportation back to the facility will be in accordance with the Mutual Aid Agreement for transfer of patents. Under most conditions, patients transferred to another acute care facility will be brought back, unless specifically requested by the receiving facility.

Staging Area Personnel

Receiving Patients

▸ **Staging Area Nurse:** coordinates and documents patients received by pre-hospital transport service, check-off master transfer sheet.

▸ **Medical Records:** checks for current MARs and assembles chart with receiving facility records.

▸ **Patient Registrar:** registers patients with information faxed from receiving facility.

▸ **Floor Nurse:** contacts units to place patients and gives information to patient registrar.

▸ **Ambulance Representative:** provides communication between Emergency Department and ambulances en route, with estimated time of arrival.

Evacuation Routes

As previously stated, in the event the hospital must be evacuated, the Hospital President (or designee) will advise as to location and routes – usually local EOC or ambulance provider routes. The primary evacuation routes will be used when evacuating to another hospital. The secondary route will be used if the primary is rendered impassable.

Receiving Patients From Other Facilities

Admission clerks will admit patients transferred from other facilities at the patient's bedside in coordination with the nursing staff on the units to which the patient is admitted. Patients will then be admitted per the standard registration process.

The facility will stock such supplies as food, water and medical supplies to adequately accommodate incoming patients. If need be, Mutual Aid Agreements and vendor contracts will be activated.

Sheltering

When the hospital accepts patients from an evacuating hospital, they will be considered inpatients. Provisions will be made for basic sustenance and medical needs of these patients.

The Hospital's Incident Commander is responsible for notifying AHCA as soon as possible, should the hospital exceed its licensed capacity.

All patients that are considered inpatients are tracked through Bed Control and the Census Summary Lists. All sheltered patients are placed on a Disaster Census List and backed up with a manual list.

Patients arriving from an evacuating facility will be admitted to the hospital via the standard admission policies unless specifically designated as sheltered patients. Patients who are considered an inpatient at another facility and transferred with that status will be evaluated on arrival for medical condition and placed in the appropriate unit per admission policy.

Non-hospitalized patients

Evacuations depend on mobility. People with physical, sensory, chronic, behavioral or cognitive disabilities may not be mobile enough for evacuations. Planners must consider the transportation needs of the community in evacuation plans. Those with disabilities that decrease their mobility may need additional help.

Preparedness

Know your community. It is important to know who might need additional services. Planners must also know where they are located within the community. Important steps of preparedness include:

- ▸ Identifying the location and condition of those with special transportation concerns;
- ▸ Identifying the type of transport necessary;
- ▸ Determining who will transport each person; and
- ▸ Identifying the equipment needed to enable transport. Door-to-door pick up may be an option.

Include community resources. Planners may benefit from using resources already in the community. Potential partners include:

- ▸ Transportation providers
- ▸ Emergency response organizations
- ▸ Local community-based services
- ▸ Advocacy groups
- ▸ Agencies that serve transportation-dependent populations
- ▸ Employment and training providers
- ▸ Health and social services, including home health care and long-term care facilities
- ▸ Faith-based organizations, including the Salvation Army
- ▸ American Red Cross
- ▸ State Departments of Transportation
- ▸ **Paratransit services:** These organizations transport those with specific mobility needs daily. Vehicles are equipped to move those with disabilities, and drivers know where their clients live. Paratransit rider lists will help emergency personnel identify those who need extra help. These can also be a communication resource.

Case Study: During Hurricane Katrina, Louisiana churches started a program called Operation Brother's Keeper. This program helped evacuate those who lacked transportation. The churches matched those who had "empty seats" in their vehicles to those who needed a ride. As a long-term goal, the program sought to relieve some of the pressures on public transit services during an evacuation. Although only a pilot program, Operation Brother's Keeper evacuated 60 percent of Jefferson Parish's population that did not have their own rides.

Lesson Learned: By partnering with private, nonprofit or faith-based groups, planners can provide additional transportation resources to those in need.

Track the whereabouts of evacuees. Keeping track of who has been evacuated, and to where, helps an evacuation run smoothly.

Emergency Shelter Medical Operations Guidelines

General Public Shelter

General public shelters are intended as safe havens for individuals and families who have been forced to leave their homes either due to an impending disaster or for short-term emergency shelter after a disaster. General public shelters remain operational until evacuees can either return home or locate alternative safe housing.

General public shelters accept people with minor injuries or illnesses, or those with physical or emotional limitations, who do not require close monitoring, assistance or equipment. Evacuees requiring skilled health or personal care will be referred to an appropriate health care facility or to a medical treatment unit/temporary infirmary. General public shelters cannot guarantee that there will be adequate medical or personal care staff or the necessary supplies or equipment for people who require such support.

Medical Treatment Unit/Temporary Infirmary/Special Needs Shelters

Medical treatment units are shelters intended to provide, to the extent practicable under emergency conditions, an environment in which medically fragile evacuees' current levels of health can be sustained. These facilities are staffed and supplied by the transferring agency and/or local health authorities and are administered by appropriate local governmental agencies in collaboration with the Red Cross or other sheltering agencies. Temporary infirmaries are portions of general public shelters intended to provide the same services. Local health authorities should determine the maximum population of medically fragile individuals that can be safely cared for in temporary infirmaries, and develop plans to open separate medical treatment units/shelters when the number of patients exceeds the capability of the public shelter temporary infirmary.

Individuals who should be directed to a medical treatment unit or temporary infirmary for care include the following:

▸ People who require assistance with medical care or treatments, such as routine injections, IV therapy, wound care, in-dwelling drainage or feeding tubes, respiratory hygiene or who are dependent upon electrical medical devices.

▸ People who are unable to care for themselves and require personal care assistance for activities of daily living (ADLs) and do not have a caregiver present, or those whose mental status requires continuous monitoring and/or a secure environment.

Medical Treatment Unit/Temporary Infirmary Site Selection

Note: This is generally a county process not a hospital function.

Selection Process

When selecting sites appropriate for use as medical treatment units/temporary infirmaries, local government should work in conjunction with specific local and private agencies to ensure that medical, health, safety and other concerns are met. Representatives from the local health department, local emergency management, local school board(s), county/municipal engineering, building inspection, American Red Cross (ARC) and voluntary agencies should all participate in the site-selection process.

Selected facilities should be (to the extent possible) compliant with the Americans with Disabilities Act (ADA), as this enables evacuees to be less dependent on staff and caregivers. Ramps, railings, easy-open doors, and lowered water fountains and wash-basins, all assist the mobility-impaired to be more independent. All public buildings should be ADA compliant.

Many states have formed Care and Shelter Technical Assistance Teams to provide technical guidance and expertise to local governments concerning care and shelter requirements and responsibilities. For more information, local government is encouraged to contact the team assigned to their area.

Selection Criteria

The primary difference in requirements between general public shelters and medical treatment units/temporary infirmaries is the need for space for sleeping, medical equipment, medical supplies and medical treatment areas, etc. Although the American Red Cross has established guidelines for selecting general public shelter sites, they do not address medical needs. However, local government, in conjunction with the ARC, should consider the following additional medical criteria:

▸ Sleeping/living space for medically fragile individuals should be calculated at approximately 60 - 80 sq. ft. per person to accommodate a 6' x 3' cot/mattress and a two-three-foot-wide perimeter.

▸ Extra space should be allocated for main aisle ways and should be wide enough to accommodate wheelchairs.

▸ Include space for two or three private examination rooms/areas.

▸ Pantry or storage space will be required for supplies.

▸ Refrigeration storage space will be required for certain pharmaceutical supplies.

▸ Water and sanitation systems should be in place and functioning.

▸ Adequate ongoing and backup electrical power should be available.

▸ Each facility to be utilized as a medical treatment unit/temporary infirmary should be identified in the local emergency plan as having priority for restoration of electrical power by power suppliers.

▸ Should have reliable onsite emergency power. Generators should be sized to fully accommodate all anticipated load requirements when the facility is fully staffed and functioning, independent of commercial electric power. Generators should have at least a 72-hour fuel supply.

Staffing The Medical Treatment Unit/Temporary Infirmary

The following staffing recommendations are intended to provide evacuees with the minimum level of care.

Standards

▸   Medical/health professionals should only perform those duties consistent with their level of expertise and only according to their professional licensure/certification and allowable scope of practice.

Staffing Schedules

▸   Staff should not be scheduled to work for more than 12 hours in a 24-hour period.

Staffing Patterns

▸   The staffing pattern should be adjusted based on the actual number and needs of the medically fragile evacuees in the medical treatment unit/temporary infirmary.

Staffing Levels and Roles

Medical Management

▸   An EMS Medical Director, Health Officer, or other designated medical manager or administrator should be available to provide overall medical management.

Physician Services

▸   A physician should be onsite.

Nursing Services

▸   A Registered Nurse should be onsite to provide supervision and direction to caregivers.

Caregivers

▸   Experienced caregivers include licensed and certified nursing staff, home health aides, paramedics, emergency medical technicians, medical/nursing students/trainees, personal care attendants, nursing aides and orderlies.

▸   Families of medically fragile evacuees should be allowed to stay with patients in the medical treatment unit/temporary infirmary, as they provide moral support and are often trained as caregivers.

Mental Health Professionals

▸   Mental health professionals capable of intervention and crisis counseling should be onsite.

Volunteers

▸   The Red Cross encourages the recruitment of volunteers to assist with non-specialized tasks.

▸   Chaplains.

Staff-to-Patient Ratios

The staff-to-patient (medically fragile evacuee) ratios are recommended only as general guidance for planning purposes and should not be construed as mandatory. Furthermore, these ratios do not imply or guarantee that any jurisdiction has the available personnel resources, either employed or voluntary, to be able to staff medical treatment units/temporary infirmaries at the recommended levels. The acuity of the population or other factors may justify an increase or decrease in the type and number of staff present.

Medical/Health Staffing	Shelter Population				
	35-40	41-80	81-120	121-160	161-200
Medical Director	1	1	1	1	1
Physician	1	2	3	4	4
RN Supervisor	1	1	1	1	1
RN/LVN	1	2	3	4	5
Experienced Caregiver	3	6	6	12	15
Mental Health	1	2	2	2	3
Total	8	14	16	24	29

Note: In addition, consider chaplains and other helpers. You will need people to move baggage, to hold sheets up while adult diapers are changed, help lift patients to prevent bed sores and so on.

Staffing Resources

Establish A Resource Directory

Develop a list of resources for medical personnel. Agencies with similar staffing resources which may be accessed include:

- local service providers to the aging
- home health agencies
- medical offices and clinics
- occupational health agencies
- managed care organizations
- ambulance companies
- hospitals and nursing homes
- nursing registries

When local staffing is unavailable, additional staff may be obtained through the State Emergency Management System.

Compensation, Reimbursement And Other Expenses

Impacted counties must be prepared to pay for all costs associated with requests for emergency medical personnel. Personnel obtained from outside the area may also incur extra costs including travel and per diem expenses.

Medical Supplies

Identify Supply Needs

A listing of suggested medical and general supplies necessary for establishing a medical treatment unit/temporary infirmary is included at the back of this document. Local government should review the suggested supply list and adopt or modify it as necessary to meet the needs of the county.

Develop a Resource Directory

▸ Maintain a resource directory with 24-hour emergency telephone numbers of vendors, suppliers, etc., and update it periodically.

▸ Develop contracts with local vendors, suppliers and/or distributors to provide the variety and quantity of supplies needed, including re-supply.

▸ When local supplies are exhausted, additional resources may be obtained through the State Emergency Management System.

Logistical Needs

▸ Determine transportation and delivery methods.

▸ Determine storage and warehousing requirements.

▸ Determine the disposition of unused supplies following the emergency.

Financial Responsibility

Impacted counties must be prepared to pay for all costs associated with requests for emergency medical supplies and equipment.

Obtaining Additional Assistance

Develop Cooperative Agreements

In coordination with the Regional Disaster Medical Health Coordinator (RDMHC), all counties within the Office of Emergency Services (OES) mutual aid region should establish regional medical and health cooperative agreements. These agreements will help provide medical and health resources when local resources are depleted. Cooperative agreements document and establish procedures for the requisition, provision and payment of medical/health resources during an emergency.

Requesting Resources

When local medical/health resources are depleted, contact the county's Medical/Health Coordinator at the Operational Area Emergency Operations Center. The Medical/Health Coordinator can assist you in locating necessary resources from elsewhere within in the county, or request assistance from the region. The Regional Disaster Medical Health Coordinator (RDMHC) will activate any regional cooperative agreements that may be in place and/or identify and coordinate resources from within the region, or, if necessary, request assistance from the state.

Training

Training, Desktop Exercises, Evaluation and Constant Revisions

An exercise is an activity designed to simulate an organization's emergency response environment and to test the effectiveness of its disaster plan. Exercises provide excellent opportunities for staff to practice new or less frequently used skills/knowledge and to integrate with other response elements in the performance of their disaster roles. Exercises measure the ability of staff to respond to unusual events and to perform in an effective and predictable manner.

Exercises are the preferred method of testing an organization's disaster response plan - before an emergency occurs. A well-executed exercise will reveal predictable flaws in the plan during exercise play and allow ample time to make necessary adjustments.

Well-planned exercises, along with appropriate follow-ups, increase readiness, build team spirit and promote confidence among staff.

The four levels of exercises are characterized below:

- Drill
  - Are usually single-function.
  - Test a trained activity.
  - Provide the building blocks of needed skills.
  - Are based upon standard procedures.
- Table-tops
  - Provide orientation and overview.
  - Involve collective problem solving.
  - Are scenario-driven.
  - Are methodical with fewer objectives.
  - Are valuable tools for learning about problem areas.
- Functional
  - Are scenario-driven.
  - Involve many objectives.
  - Are usually conducted in "real time."
  - Use simulators to provide realism for participants.

      ▷ Are command post and EOC focused.

      ▷ Are management-oriented.

▸ Full-scale

      ▷ Are driven by a well-developed scenario.

      ▷ Involve many objectives on all levels of response.

      ▷ Simulate actual disaster events.

      ▷ Involve "real time" players and equipment.

      ▷ Contain special effects that add to realism (i.e., moulage, participant behaviors, rubble, etc.).

      ▷ Require the highest level of training, organization, coordination and planning.

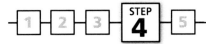

STEP 4
Transportation

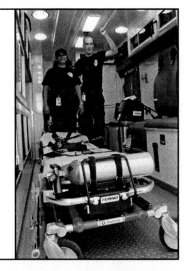

Transportation needs will differ dependent upon the type of emergency. Arrangements should be made for the following means of transportation to be available – depending on local weather conditions:

▸ Employee Shuttle Busses

▸ Patient Transport Vehicles

▸ Facility Motor Pool

▸ Volunteer Motorized Boats

▸ County, State and National Guard Vehicles

▸ Ambulances

▸ Snow Skis

Transportation for Essential Personnel

The Transportation Supervisor should coordinate picking up individuals designated as Essential Personnel for the emergency at hand, if the individuals cannot provide their own transportation and if road conditions allow. If essential personnel are likely to remain at the facility for some days, for example, because of a severe weather event, they should bring in the own personal supplies. A suggested list would be:

Checklist

☐ Food (non-perishable)

☐ Water (at least one gallon per person, per day)

☐ Blankets, pillows, sheets

☐ Air mattress

☐ Flashlight, batteries, extra bulbs

☐ Medications (seven-day supply of prescription medications)

☐ Reading materials, playing cards

☐ Toiletries

☐ Extra clothes (shorts, tennis shoes)

☐ Plastic bags

☐ Portable radio or small battery-powered TV

☐ Pocket change (quarters and small bills)

☐ Several changes of work clothes

Keep track of transportation resources. In an emergency, resources will be limited. Communities should prioritize transportation for those with impaired mobility. Planners should keep a sharp eye on the transportation resources they have available and the needs of the community. Consider the following:

▸ Maintain a list of transportation resources.

▸ Organize it by type and availability.

▸ Also include things such as vehicle accessibility and capacity.

Develop lists of additional resources. Consider fuel needs, access to vehicles, mileage to be traveled and storage of resources. Keep all lists up-to-date before, during, and after an event.

🔘 Must Do ━━━━━━━━

Keep transportation records. During an evacuation, it is likely that people will be scattered. Friends and family may be separated.

Crosswalk plans with neighboring communities. Ensure that your plans do not rely on the same equipment as a neighboring community. A single transport agency may have multiple contracts for their resources. When disaster strikes, there may not be enough vehicles or drivers to meet all of the agreements. Planners should create back up plans for limited resources.

Provide specialized transportation equipment. According to U.S. DOT's Catastrophic Hurricane Evacuation Plan Evaluation, "even in urban areas where more modes [of transportation] are available, few plans recognize the potential role for intercity buses, trains, airplanes and boats. These modes may be particularly important for persons who cannot evacuate in personal vehicles including persons with various disabilities." Planners might look to include such resources in their plans. They might also incorporate:

- School buses
- Wheelchair accessible school buses
- Private vehicles, like sedans or minivans
- Private medical transport vehicles

Some people may have serious medical conditions that need immediate attention. They will need to be transported as quickly as possible. Consider using life-flight helicopters or MICU ambulances. Some equipment must be operated by trained personnel. Planners should keep a master list of drivers by status and availability. This will help match the appropriate equipment and driver skill level in an emergency.

Review emergency transportation plans. Emergency responders and volunteers should be familiar with emergency plans. The emergency planner can help this process. Additionally, planners can help train and review how to transport those with disabilities. Include ways to transport service animals.

Response

Use appropriate vehicles for transport. Individuals with disabilities will have a diverse set of needs. Not everyone will need specialized transportation equipment. Many will need assistance. For example, those with vision impairment, mental retardation or psychiatric disorders will be able to ride in any type of transportation. Those that require assistants will benefit if assistants travel with them in the same vehicle. People in wheelchairs will require special vans with lifts for transportation. Others who use mobility aids may need vehicles with enough room for their special equipment.

Planners should consider the range of equipment available for transport. They should also consider how to best maximize those resources.

Provide door-to-door service. Consider providing door-to-door services in an evacuation. This will be especially helpful for those who have mobility limitations or do not have their own transportation. Local organizations, such as Meals-on-Wheels or faith-based groups, can help. These organizations maintain lists of those that need door-to-door pick-up. They may even have the resources to help evacuate.

For people with disabilities, separation from a caregiver or support network can cause problems. Transportation operators can create rosters to record service. These billing rosters will help recover revenue. It may also help friends and families track the whereabouts of their loved ones. A roster should contain the following information:

▸ Name of driver

▸ Driver's telephone number

▸ Time departed staging area

▸ Time arrived at sheltering location

▸ Vehicle number

▸ Sheltering location

▸ Person(s) transported

Case Study: During the evacuations in Hurricane Katrina, victims were poorly tracked. Once they reached their destination, some evacuees were unable to contact their families. Others were separated from their groups during the evacuation. Family members loading on different buses thought that all the buses were going to the same destination when they were not. Once phone and Internet service was restored, family and friends began filing missing person reports with groups such as the American Red Cross. Other tools to assist in locating missing people began operations including the "Katrina People Finder Project" and Web boards such as the "Yahoo! Message board Katrina: Search for Missing People." Some of the more successful tracking was done by The National Center for Missing & Exploited Children (NCMEC). This group staffed a hotline to take reports of missing and found children and adults.

Lesson Learned: Communities may benefit from having centralized hotlines or message boards. This will help families locate each other following an evacuation. Ensure that people with disabilities can access the systems, and advertise the system before and during the evacuation.

Finding transportation resources may be difficult. Drivers may be stranded, burned out or gone. During Hurricane Floyd in 1999, some drivers were sent out to deliver urgently needed supplies but became stranded because of the storm. As drivers, they were no longer available and the supplies didn't get through. Plan accordingly.

The whole community may be competing for the same resources, including fuel. Private owners may want vehicles returned, so they can begin their own recovery. Individuals with disabilities may need a certain type of vehicle for transport. Logically, these resources may be in high demand.

Arrange to return people home, based on their needs. Returning to an area following a disaster is likely to be a slow process. Long-term contracts with transport services may be needed. Damages may require long stays in shelters or other disaster housing. Regardless, people may be eager to return to their homes. This will place limited transportation resources in high demand. Planners may work to schedule transportation back to a home or community in shifts. Individuals with disabilities may have a greater need to return to their home or care facility. Planners should prioritize the transport of individuals in need to ease the burden that a disaster may cause.

Special arrangements will have to be made with law enforcement to allow staff to get to and from work in the event of a curfew being imposed.

Ensure transportation is accessible. Even during the recovery phase, transportation will be in high demand. This demand will likely outpace resources. It is important to keep transport services accessible to everyone in the community.

▸ Prioritize specialized vehicles for those who require them.

▸ Passengers may require door-to-door drop off or assistance entering the home. Plan to have transportation providers give this aid.

▸ Accessibility may be affected by a disaster. For example, someone's home may remain unaffected, but their ramp may be damaged. Include this information in post-disaster assessment.

Transportation and Emergency Preparedness Checklist

From the events of September 11, 2001, to the devastation wrought by recent hurricanes in Florida and all along the Gulf Coast, the manner in which plans, procedures and responses to emergency events are implemented, clearly can save lives and rebuild communities. The need to safely and efficiently transport people, particularly those for whom community and public transportation is their primary means of mobility, before, during and after emergency situations, is a crucial consideration.

The Transportation and Emergency Preparedness Checklist was developed by a gathering of public and community transportation professionals who convened in April 2006 at the behest of the National Consortium on the Coordination of Human Service Transportation. It is intended to provide practical guidance to transportation providers and their partner organizations in planning for the transport of persons requiring mobility assistance in the event of an emergency. The Checklist was designed to be used as a tool during the planning process, prior to an emergency situation, to ensure safe and appropriate transportation for transportation-dependent populations, including older adults, persons living in group situations, persons with disabilities (including persons with physical, visual, hearing, intellectual, psychiatric, learning and cognitive disabilities), and individuals without access to personal transportation.

Planning and Coordination Before Emergency Situations

Establish and maintain working relationships with partner organizations including a variety of community-based organizations, including advocacy organizations, agencies that serve the transportation-dependent populations, employment and training providers, health and human service agencies, faith and community-based organizations, departments of Workforce Development and

One-Stop Career Center, and emergency response organizations and personnel. Maintain an up-to-date contact list and network of communication.

Organize and conduct regular, periodic drills that include the procedures for evacuating transportation-dependent populations.

Clarify rules, regulations and chains of responsibility at the local, state and federal levels.

Identify Those Needing Transportation Assistance

▸ Collaborate with partner organizations in identifying individuals who may require transportation assistance in the event of an emergency.

▸ In accordance with Health Insurance Portability and Accountability Act (HIPAA) regulations, explore the development of voluntary registries for individuals requiring transportation assistance. For those individuals agreeing to be on voluntary registries, seek to have a signed authorization. Further information on signed authorizations is available through www.hhs.gov/ocr/hipaa/decisiontool/tool/auths.html.

▸ Identify and determine the appropriate transportation response for persons unable to reach a pick-up/drop-off location or staging area on their own, what entity will handle such needs, and what types of vehicles/equipment will be required.

▸ Determine strategies for tracking individuals who are evacuated. Information should include the passenger's name, point of origin, departure time, final destination and arrival time. Ensure that enough transportation capacity exists with transportation providers, partner agencies and suppliers to effectively meet the demand in an emergency.

Public Involvement and Community Outreach

▸ Conduct outreach and education that ensures public awareness of the transportation plan, particularly as it relates to those populations requiring transportation assistance in the event of an emergency.

▸ Include members of the public and private sector (including local businesses) in the planning and outreach process, ensuring participation of potentially transportation-dependent populations including older adults, persons with disabilities (including physical, visual, hearing, intellectual, psychiatric, learning and cognitive disabilities), people living in group situations and those without access to personal transportation.

▸ Using a variety of media and accessible formats such as Braille, large-type, audio and appropriate languages, broadly publicize information related to staging areas and pick-up/drop-off locations. Determine a point-of-contact person who will address questions from the public.

▸ Provide information in a variety of formats to accommodate non-English speakers and persons with visual or auditory disabilities or difficulties reading printed text due to visual impairments, color blindness, illiteracy, learning disabilities or mobility limitations that may interfere with holding or turning the pages of printed materials.

Equipment and Personnel Support

▸ Establish a reliable communications system utilizing available technologies. Ensure the availability of an alternative system in the event that normal dispatching networks and telephones are not functional and when electrical power may be out.

▸ Maintain a transportation resources list by type and availability, including vehicle accessibility and capacity information. Develop procedures for the acquisition of additional accessible transportation equipment, securement devices, supplies and resources.

▸ Secure agreements with fuel suppliers and other local agencies (such as police and fire departments) that require a reliable fuel source. Distribute and maintain list of these fueling sites.

▸ Compile and distribute evacuation route information to be used during emergency operations, including alternative evacuation route information should the primary route be inaccessible due to damage or danger.

▸ Provide staff training regarding the emergency plan, including a review of procedures for transporting persons with a variety of assistance needs, as well as the transport of service animals.

▸ Identify staff with foreign language and sign language skills; provide staff training to ensure basic communication skills in sign language and relevant foreign languages.

▸ Maintain a master list of drivers by status and availability.

▸ Prior to activation, provide staff the opportunity to ensure the safety and security of their loved ones and personal property.

When an Emergency is Imminent

▸ Local officials notify partner agencies and organizations of threat.

▸ Following agreed-upon plans, coordination begins among emergency departments, public safety agencies, hospitals, transportation providers, etc.

▸ Designated transportation staging areas and pick-up/drop-off locations are activated.

▸ Staff, key partner agencies and other vital personnel as designated in the emergency plan are placed on stand-by.

▸ All drivers and operations personnel are notified of potential deployment of emergency plan, and are instructed to follow their pre-determined emergency preparation roles.

▸ Following established protocols, persons with assistance needs who require direct personal contact are notified of the impending evacuation and where they will be transported.

▸ All passengers are transported to their destinations on the planned evacuation routes or alternative routes, as necessary.

During Emergency Situations

▸ Evacuation notifications are communicated to partner organizations, and, following established protocols, to pre-determined transportation-dependent groups such as older adults, persons living in group situations, persons with disabilities (including persons with physical, visual, hearing, intellectual, psychiatric, learning and cognitive disabilities) and individuals without access to personal transportation.

▸ In accordance with the local plan, participating agencies and organizations are involved with necessary personnel to affect evacuation, sheltering, response and initial recovery.

▸ Emergency transportation officials report to Emergency Operations Center (EOC).

▸ Transportation service is activated upon request of EOC officials, or as stipulated in the plan.

▸ All transportation activities and operations are coordinated from the EOC.

▸ Transportation operations are directed over normal dispatching networks (if available), telephones (landlines) and cell phones, or previously tested and agreed-upon alternative communications systems, as necessary.

▸ Personnel and equipment are deployed to pre-assigned locations or staging areas, including designated supervisors, mechanics and drivers.

▸ Vehicles are fueled prior to evacuation, refueled as necessary during the evacuation process, fueled after the final trip to the sheltering location, and then taken to the pre-determined location where they will be housed safely until the response effort begins.

▸ When a vehicle reaches full capacity, the driver departs to the designated evacuation location.

▸ Door-to-door service is provided as designated in the emergency plan, based upon medical necessity or the specific transportation needs of the passenger.

▸ A roster is prepared and maintained by the operator, containing at a minimum the following information:

  ▹ Name of driver
  ▹ Driver's telephone number
  ▹ Time departed staging area
  ▹ Time arrived at sheltering location
  ▹ Vehicle number
  ▹ Sheltering location
  ▹ Trip mileage

This roster is vital, as it provides a record of service that can be used after the emergency for billing purposes.

▸   As highlighted in the emergency response training, the operator reports to transportation supervisors at the agreed-upon location to receive further instructions. Operators shall continue transporting until released by the EOC.

▸   In the event the EOC must be evacuated, transportation officials will provide vehicles to transport EOC personnel and essential equipment to pre-designated alternative EOC locations.

Reentry and Recovery Preparations

▸   Initiate recovery operations as designated in the emergency plan.

▸   Following the plan, operators and vehicles remain at the sheltering location to return evacuees to their home communities. Generally, passengers will return with the same operator and via the same vehicle used during the evacuation. Alternative plans for return should be in place, in the event that the evacuation lasts for days, weeks or possibly longer.

▸   Operators and passengers have picture identification to get back to their home area.

▸   All operators will remain on duty in accordance with the emergency plan.

▸   Transportation officials, in coordination with the EOC, will assign other tasks relating to the transportation component of reentry and recovery as the situation dictates.

▸   Vehicles will return to established drop-off points near passengers' residences or directly to the residence, based upon necessity.

Assessment

▸   Evaluate emergency response effort, identifying successes and gaps in service.

▸   Make appropriate changes to the emergency plan, and communicate such changes to partner organizations and the public.

Additional Resources

Are You Ready? A Guide to Citizen Preparedness, FEMA www.citizencorps.gov/ready/cc_pubs.shtm

Assisting People with Disabilities in a Disaster, FEMA www.fema.gov/plan/prepare/specialplans.shtm

Catastrophic Hurricane Evacuation Plan Evaluation, U.S. Department of Transportation
www.fhwa.dot.gov/reports/hurricanevacuation/

Disaster Mitigation and Persons with Disabilities, Independent Living Resource Utilization
www.ilru.org/html/training/webcasts/handouts/2003/08-27-PB/Transcript.txt

Disaster Preparedness and People with Disabilities or Special Health Care Needs, Iowa's Early and Periodic Screening, Diagnosis and Treatment Program (EPSDT)
www.iowaepsdt.org/EPSDTNews/2002/win02/disaster.htm

Disaster Preparedness: Reasoning WHY Physical, Emotional and Financial Preparation for Disabled Citizens, How Eliminating Limited Perceptions Unifies Us (HELPU Fire and Life Safety)
www.helpusafety.org/3PREPSDI.pdf

Drivewell, American Society on Aging
www.asaging.org/asav2/drivewell/index.cfm?CFID=23210127&CFTOKEN=62971471

Emergency Preparation and Evacuation for Employees with Disabilities: Identifying Potential Interventions and Methods for Testing Them, Glen W. White, PhD
www2.ku.edu/~rrtcpbs/powerpoint/EPEED.ppt

Emergency Preparation and People with Disabilities, National Service Inclusion Project, National Council on Disability (NCD) www.serviceandinclusion.org/index.php?page=emergency

Emergency Tip Sheets for People with Disabilities, Independent Living Resource Center of San Francisco www.prepare.org/disabilities/disabilities.htm

Evacuation issues for people with disabilities, National Council on Disability (NCD)
hwww.tvworldwide.com/events/NOD/player.cfm

Last Invited In, Forced to be Last Out, Illinois Assistive Technology Project
www.iltech.org/erevac.asp

Orientation Manual for First Responders on the Evacuation of Persons with Disabilities, FEMA
www.usfa.dhs.gov/downloads/pdf/publications/FA-235-508.pdf

Preparing for Emergencies: A Checklist for People with Mobility Problems, FEMA
www.montgomerycountymd.gov/Content/homelandsecurity/preparedness/mobilitychecklist.pdf

Report on SNAKE Project, National Organization on Disability
www.nod.org/Resources/PDFs/katrina_snake_report.pdf (PDF - 56 KB)

Special Needs Planning Considerations for Services and Support Providers, FEMA
training.fema.gov/EMIWeb/IS/IS197SP.asp

Strategies in Emergency Preparedness for Transportation-Dependent Populations, National Consortium on Human Services Transportation www.dotcr.ost.dot.gov/Documents/Emergency/Emergency%20Preparedness%20Strategy%20Paper.doc

The Emergency Preparedness Initiative (EPI) Guide for Emergency Managers, Planners & Responders, National Organization on Disability
www.nod.org/resources/PDFs/epiguide2005.pdf (PDF - 165 KB)

Transportation and Emergency Preparedness Checklist, National Consortium on the Coordination of Human Service Transportation www.dotcr.ost.dot.gov/Documents/Emergency/Emergency%20Checklist.doc

Working Conference on Emergency Management and People with Disabilities and the Elderly
www.add-em-conf.com/presentations.htm

Patient Critical Evacuation Information Tracking Form

Blank Forms are available online. Please see Table of Contents for instructions.

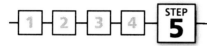

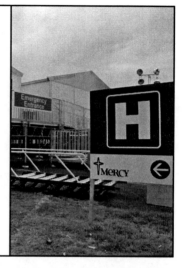

STEP 5

Recovery

In the event the facility's normal operations have been interrupted as a result of an emergency situation, departments must have a pre-established plan for returning to normal operations. This will include areas such as:

▸ Information Services restoring data from offsite storage locations.

▸ Finance and having the ability to issue checks and provide cash.

▸ Environmental Services and Facilities Management for restoring areas where clean up and repair are needed.

Post-Storm Actions

Once the National Weather Service has announced that the storm has moved out of the area, clean-up operations shall begin and normal routine resumed. Employees who did not report for duty during the severe weather will be expected to report for duty immediately so that employees who have been working extended shifts may be relieved.

Department	Actions
All Departments	Begin clean-up operations and resume normal routine.
Administration and Executive Group	Collect damage reports from Facilities Management and Nursing Units.
	Maintain property damage list for insurance reporting.
	Evaluate locations for re-opening and initiate public notification through Public Affairs.
Directors and Department Managers	Initiate clean-up operations and resume normal operations.
	Report damage to Administration.
	Prepare post-storm report/critique and send to Safety/Security Administration. Include actions taken and recommendations for change.
Environmental Services	Begin clean-up operations, as necessary and where instructed by ICC.
	Assist with replacing furniture in conference rooms and dining areas.
	Return any army cots to warehouse.
Facilities Management	When instructed by ICC, make a survey of buildings and grounds to determine and document storm damage with video and note-taking.
	Use Extreme Caution When Entering Or Working Near Structures That May Have Been Damaged Or Weakened By Severe Weather, As They May Collapse Without Warning.
	Be observant for gas leaks. DO NOT take any ignition sources such as cigarettes or torches into damaged areas.
	Be observant for damaged electrical lines or short circuits. Stay away from fallen wires and wet electrical equipment. Wear rubber-soled boots/shoes to prevent shock hazards.
	Report survey findings to ICC.
Food Services	Begin departmental clean-up operations.
	Make plans to utilize emergency supplies.
Guest Services	Report to nursing units to assist with returning patients to their rooms and to assist with clean-up operations.
Nursing Services	Report physical damage and number of rooms uninhabitable to ICC.
	Return patients to their rooms if rooms are not damaged. Maintain temporary rest areas until patients can be transferred to other rooms.
Security	Resume routine post assignments.
	Make rounds in and around all areas for possible looting activity.
Service Center	Disband Personnel Pool once clean-up operations are complete.

Repopulation after Evacuation

An evacuation of a general acute care hospital impatient building occurs following an incident or series of incidents that result in a situation which is, or may become, detrimental to the well-being of patients, staff, workers or visitors in the hospital.

Any evacuation of a hospital building should be implemented in accordance with the facility's Emergency Plan as well as in coordination with Operational Area Disaster and Emergency Management Plan(s). Evacuations can consist of the following scenarios:

▸ Full evacuation of the hospital campus

▸ Full evacuation of one or more inpatient care buildings on campus

▸ Partial evacuation of one or more inpatient care buildings

Buildings that house inpatients who are released or transferred to make room to receive inpatients evacuated from other inpatient care buildings are not considered buildings that experienced an evacuation. However, program flexibility may be required from the L&C district office to treat patients in these buildings.

An evacuation can be voluntary or mandatory. A voluntary evacuation decision is made by the Chief Executive Officer (CEO) or Incident Commander (IC) and is based on the hospital's EOP and available internal and external information. A mandatory evacuation is an evacuation that is ordered by an authorized governmental authority having jurisdiction. Government authorities with jurisdiction include, but are not limited to, fire, law enforcement, OSHPD and local emergency services.

A hospital may be able to remain operational and/or avoid voluntary evacuation by seeking program flexibility from the appropriate L&C district office. For example, for a partial evacuation, the hospital may be able to move inpatients from damaged units by expanding capacity in operational inpatient units or maintain limited operations by the use of alternate treatment areas while preparing evacuated areas for repopulation. Recovery and repopulation of evacuated facilities should be included in hospital preparedness activities and its EP. Steps taken prior to, or at the time of evacuation, will facilitate more efficient repopulation of facilities, for example:

▸ Report partial or full evacuation to district office, Operational Area Office of Emergency Services (OES) and the Local Emergency Medical Services Agency and other agencies, as appropriate.

▸ Maintain surveillance monitoring of temperatures, refrigeration, air/water quality, pharmaceuticals and facility security, as feasible.

The hospital CEO, his/her designee, or the IC has the ultimate responsibility to ensure a safe environment for patients, staff and visitors. In making a decision to evacuate or repopulate, the CEO or IC should use the Hospital Incident Command System (HICS) and, in doing so, give consideration to consulting with key departments, the chief of the medical staff, the local department of health, and other public safety and utility agencies, as appropriate.

Also, the CEO or IC will:

▸ Give consideration to whether an evacuation may be more harmful to the patients, staff and visitors than sheltering in place. Consult with appropriate hospital departments and external agencies in making a determination regarding whether the facility has adequate resources and is clean, sanitary and safe to repopulate and/or receive patients after an evacuation. Each decision shall be considered on a case-by-case basis. It is understood that an evacuated hospital/ building will not be staffed, nor will perishable resources be re-stocked until necessary approvals are received and repopulation plans are initiated.

▸ Base the decision of whether to repopulate on the merits of the evacuated area alone and not be biased by the argument that returning to the evacuated area is better than where patients are currently located. Whether patients need to move from their current temporary location is a separate issue. An alternate temporary location may be more appropriate than repopulating them in an evacuated building.

▸ Be aware that any evacuation is considered a reportable event.

Mitigation

> After any event, planners should identify lessons learned and ways to improve.

Draft an After-Action Report. Planners should create an after-action report. This will help evaluate response and recovery from an event. It will also help identify successes and gaps in service. This will help improve future operations. Involving partners in the feedback is critical to successfully reviewing and improving on the plan. Consider using community partner workshops, meetings, driver reports, etc., to gather information. Also use Incident Action Plans, activity logs, and functional and position checklists.

Clarify the Evacuation Process. Planners should look for ways to make evacuation transport services more well-known. For example, a signage committee can examine what signs are needed at the pick-up and drop-off points. Better signs can help traffic and pedestrian flow. They can also increase the efficiency and safety of an evacuation. This will be particularly important for individuals with disabilities who may take longer to evacuate.

Major Damage

Section 130025 (a) of the Health and Safety Code states, "In the event of a seismic event, or other natural or manmade calamity that the office believes is of a magnitude so that it may have compromised the structural integrity of a hospital building, or any major system of a hospital building, the office shall send one or more authorized representatives to examine the structure or system. "System" for these purposes shall include, but not be limited to, the electrical, mechanical, plumbing, and fire and life safety system of the hospital building. If, in the opinion of the office, the structural integrity of the hospital building or any system has been compromised and damaged to a degree that the hospital building has been made unsafe to occupy, the office may cause to be placed on the hospital building either a red tag, a yellow tag or a green tag."

A hospital building with a red tag (unsafe) or a yellow tag (restricted access) cannot be repopulated until the tag is removed. A green tag indicates that the building is safe for repopulation.

Hierarchy of Repopulation Approval(s)

Dependent upon circumstances, the following sequential steps should be expected prior to the repopulation of evacuated hospital facilities.

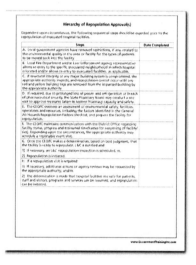

Blank Forms are available online. Please see Table of Contents for instructions.

Lightning Source UK Ltd.
Milton Keynes UK
UKOW041825111111

181913UK00002B/5/P